Freedom from Obesity
and
Sugar Addiction

Martha L. Pekarek

Published by Wheatmark™
610 East Delano Street, Suite 104, Tucson, Arizona 85705 U.S.A.
www.wheatmark.com

ISBN-10: 1-58736-694-0
ISBN-13: 978-1-58736-694-9
LCCN: 2006931652

DEDICATION

THIS BOOK IS DEDICATED to my precious daughter, Heather, who encouraged me in my efforts to lose my excess poundage and prayed that I would find the answer. She put up with my years of weight frustration and has always been my biggest supporter. She's fought the same battle at my side and given me three wonderful grandchildren to enjoy during the process. It is my hope that my grandchildren and readers will choose vibrant living foods to achieve maximum health and avoid products that bring obesity, sickness, and sadness.

Special thanks as well to both of my sisters, Marji and Mary Beth, who edited this book while pursuing extraordinary lives of their own.

Contents

CHAPTER 1

Fat and Fifty

"We often create our own troubles."

AGE FIFTY DISAPPEARED IN my rearview mirror years ago! It's that sudden awareness of having a limited amount of tomorrows left to accomplish all of life's goals. Achieving and keeping a safe and sane weight has always been at the top of my list, but my poor eating choices resulted in obesity. Until I understood that I had a food addiction and learned how to stop its hideous hold, any serious weight loss could not be achieved.

I applaud all of you who are searching for a way to take off the unhealthy poundage and refusing to give up. Losing weight while working toward a healthy lifestyle of eating and exercise habits will prolong your life and allow you to live a more satisfying quality-filled time on this Earth. Just achieving your ideal weight will not keep you healthy if you are choosing poor quality foods. It will be next to impossible to maintain your best weight while eating things that are unfit for human consumption. Eating nutritious foods allows your entire body to function properly while you gain better health and establish control over food cravings. We now have a clearer understanding of what is causing most of us to overeat, and addictive foods are at the top of the list, including processed sugar.

1

The first and last time I went tubing (*tubing: the art of pulling an inflated flat-topped plastic thing behind a speeding powerboat*), I tumbled off the tube in the middle of an east Texas lake and found myself too bottom-heavy to pull myself back on. One of the nice relatives risked a torn shoulder and permanent back injury to heave my hulk out of the water and back onto the tube for further fun in the sun. It was either that or swim some distance to shore, which didn't seem likely since deadly poisonous moccasins (a type of water snake) bite swimmers in the nearby shoreline vegetation occasionally. Another alternative would have been for several family members to pull me back on board, in which case we may have capsized the entire lot.

When we are obese, we experience many embarrassing moments like these. I'm sure you have agonizing memories buried in your consciousness, hoping they will never surface again.

Your doctor hints that you need to drop a ridiculous number of pounds that seems impossible to achieve, so you discard that doctor because you are too embarrassed to face him again and move on to the next. In frustration, you head for the corner ice cream shop and treat yourself to the largest swirl they offer. You rationalize that you will begin your diet tomorrow.

Occasionally, you'll see someone actually lose weight and keep it off. Why can she do the impossible while you can't seem to get it together? Even the word "fat" makes you cringe. You beat yourself up mentally. You don't want to be one of those statistically 60 percent-plus of American adults who are "fat," and you certainly don't want to be obese, which by standard definition is "extremely fat" or by scientific definition is at least 20 percent or more over your perfect weight. In other words, if you weigh 150 pounds instead of the 125 you should weigh, you are considered extremely fat (obese) by life insurance standards. You are found guilty by a simple math calculation. Multiply 1.2 times the amount you should weigh ($125 \times 1.2 = 150$) in order to see where you cross the definition line at obesity. Personally speaking, finding myself at 150 pounds after hovering around 200 pounds for years seemed very respectable to me, but every extra pound does unfortunately stress body organs and joints.

Morbid obesity, sometimes defined as being more than one hundred pounds above your "normal" weight, is incompatible with health because it increases the risk of disease. Being too lean may also compromise health. Those who are somewhat overweight but physically fit may enjoy a healthier and longer old age than those who are lean and not fit.

If you're an average female in your twenties (and not an Olympic type), you should ideally have no more than 22 percent BMI (body mass index or percentage of body fat compared to other things like bone tissue). My BMI was somewhere near the bright red zone of 40 percent. Red is the color that signals danger, *danger*, DANGER, where warning sirens blare and a flight attendant prepares passengers for a "crash" scenario! Before your last rites occur, this book intends to encourage and show you how to achieve better health while losing your excess poundage, even if you have already slid over the edge of that precipice into serious afflictions.

For a quick calculated guess at your BMI percentage, go to the Web site www.mehndiskinart.com/bmi_calculator.htm. This is only a rough average estimate, as there is no way a math calculation can measure your muscle mass or bone density or fitness level. More accurate tests are done at universities by sinking you briefly into a tub of water.

By now, your intuition tells you that you need to avoid those chocolates that someone brought to work, but your taste buds scream for gratification the instant you see them. You reach for only one and then return for another and another. You are unable to stop, and you don't even know why. Why some of us are addicted to sugar or chocolate while others can easily control the amount consumed is one of life's great mysteries. A clue to addictive behavior in eating is when you begin to munch uncontrollably, shoving potato chip after potato chip into your mouth even when you know you are not hungry. This is mind-less eating and happens only when you are eating addictive foods. You can literally change your body chemistry and be-come a fat-burning machine by making adjustments to what you eat. You will not be giving up any foods that are healthy for you! Better health should be your ultimate goal; you can lose hundreds of pounds and still develop such terrible health problems from poor quality foods that you will not be able to enjoy your life or maintain your weight.

Ideally, at 5-foot, 2-inches tall, my weight—according to life insurance charts—should be somewhere between 118 to 133 pounds for a medium-framed female. I always weigh myself first thing in the morning before eating. This will most likely be your lowest weight of the day. I feel best at a weight of about 130 pounds, which I have never seen in my adult life until age fifty-five. Much below 125, my face appears sunken and I can count each individual rib. Also, too low a body mass is very difficult to maintain. The less one weighs, the fewer calories you need to maintain that weight. Over 130 pounds, my waist-line increases exponentially for every pound of fat gained. At 150 pounds, I sport a strapping 36-inch waistline. For the verti-cally-challenged (short) individual, there are fewer places for fat to hide, so girth expands outward at a phenomenal rate. With proper nutrition, I'm living proof that a dead metabolism can rev up and work properly, even in middle age.

One rather odd "time warp phenomenon" was when I weighed 156 pounds in high school over forty years ago and was considered fat by my peers. Most other teenage girls were less chunky than me. At 156 pounds forty years later, I did not "look fat" by comparison to my peers because of the increasing obesity of adults around me. By this time in my life, I was now in the minority of shrinking adults, while most other middle-aged folks were becoming increasingly heavy.

My bone structure is solid with square shoulders (I re-move those ridiculous shoulder pads in clothes or my shoulders would appear higher than my chin). I've never been one of those petite individuals able to slip bangle bracelets over wrists (my knuckles do not bend) or jump into size-four jeans. I am currently ecstatic to fit into a pair of size-nine pants with a stretchy waistband! My extreme change in sizes spiraled downward from a woman's size twenty-two.

Perhaps you have made small changes in your diet or exercise routines to correct for certain years of neglect. You may be exercising more or cutting out various foods, but the pounds persist. You find it almost impossible to give up your ice cream, cookies, or chocolates. Have you ever wondered why it's so difficult to give up something that tastes so good? Perhaps you stopped raiding the refrigerator after dinner. Maybe you've seen the sense of eating a large breakfast before beginning your active day or ceased eating three hours before bedtime. Eating a large meal before bedtime results in restless sleep. Your metabolism slows down as you sleep, so more of the calories consumed later in the evening are converted immediately to storage fat. Possibly you've resisted drinking sodas and switched to unsweetened tea. Making small corrective adjustments over a lifetime helps keep you on course. But the corrective actions haven't been enough. What then?

Desserts have become an obsessively important part of your life. You reward yourself often. You may have suffered for days without any sweets, but one bite puts you over the edge and back into the cycle of eating uncontrollably while trying to satisfy those sugar cravings.

You purchased different exercise gadgets to burn up calories, and still the pounds clung to ever-widening parts of your anatomy. You want to wear those shrinking clothes in the back of your closet and have more energy to keep up with the physically active and those who act like they are alive in a high-energy world. You purchased a new gym membership and promised yourself you would get back into that high-school size. You bought diet pills that promised you the world but left you with a racing heart or sent you running to the bathroom—and still you didn't lose an ounce. You became frustrated with yourself for wasting scarce bank funds on such foolishness. You're embarrassed to have anyone see certain parts of your flesh because of your bulging rolls of fat. By now, you may be limiting yourself to one serving of dessert per day just to keep yourself from becoming the next Boeing 737, but the serving portion might still be the entire half gallon of mint fudge ice cream.

Each day that you have not yet achieved perfection, your heart sinks into despair. After the last birthday cake with the one-inch thick, creamy icing is served and the party ends, you face the reality that you are still obese, not chubby, not pleasingly plump, but FAT! VERY FAT!

We're not discussing the extra fifteen pounds that someone gained over thirty years of selective indulgence here. We're yelling OBESE—as in adding twenty-five pounds in three months without blinking, that kind of eating. It's exhausting heaviness from carrying all that extra weight around with you everywhere. You've got a one-piece black bathing suit in your drawer that is now six sizes too small. You don't care at this point whether or not your figure attracts attention or if heads turn. You don't really care if you ever fit into tiny sizes again. You'd settle for a size fourteen at this juncture in your life because you want to be able to see your feet under your belly. You just want to weigh less, have some self-esteem, and not be exhausted climbing one flight of stairs.

You've got enough outfits that don't fit to clothe all the ladies in church. You cannot bring yourself to throw them out just yet. Trashing those outdated relics would be giving up hope for the last time and admitting total defeat. You refuse to give into the feeling of being a failure. Someday you will find the answer to what works best for you. While you struggle with your dilemma, you reach for another Reese's and wonder how you could ever live without sweets. It seems that chocolate is one of your greatest comforts in life, and it's on your mind constantly.

You buy every new diet book that appears on the market. You watch all the weight-loss television programs and religiously buy every magazine pertaining to weight loss. Someday you will grab that silver bullet of freedom, and those demons of diet hell will never taunt you again. You intensify your commitment to exercise, even though you have a history of chronic back problems. You realize with a groan that you are still battling the same old weight problem that plagued you yesterday and last year and decades before that. None of the diets worked permanently. You lost some of the weight numerous times, only to regain it all back plus more. Is dietary success for you just an illusion? Are you genetically programmed to always be fat?

Don't you believe it!

Can it possibly be that you are sabotaging yourself? Are there certain foods that trigger uncontrollable hunger and cravings? Is there a potential to lose interest in sweets so that you will never be tempted to eat them again? You may think you want to lose weight because of the kids, your significant other, or because it's more fun at the beach. In reality, you just want to lose weight to feel your best, look good, and keep it off permanently. You want to get your health back. You want your life back. You are embarrassed by shapeless square clothes that are two yards wide. You'd like to stop being physically exhausted after barely any effort.

You want the spring in your step and the dimples to show in the right places when you smile. Instead, your belly is sagging over your thighs. Your knees ache walking through the mall, and your legs and feet hurt for hours at night after being vertical all day. You're too tired to do the things you used to enjoy doing. Your back hurts. Your upper arms flap as you move, and you haven't worn a sleeveless item in years. Your shoes don't fit right, and your feet suffer from blisters, corns,

and bunions. You stop going out because you don't want to be
seen. The doctor says he needs to remove some calcium deposits that will keep you off your feet for weeks, which means
no exercise and more pounds. You make excuses for wearing
soft sandals in December. You don't remove your jacket even
when it's hot. You are ashamed of your own appearance. You
certainly don't want to run into the family member who has
never gained a pound in his entire adult life. He conjures up
his wisdom of the ages, though he has never been overweight,
and offers you his gems on weight control.

You've watched too many programs on extreme weight-
loss methods that require surgery, and you don't want to go
there. Are they nuts? Do they want to ruin their health? Don't
they realize that a small percentage die from the surgery or
from complications later? How can they spend thousands of
their own personal dollars and risk life itself for something that
should be so simple? Is it because the life of the obese person
is perceived to be a greater challenge than one can sometimes
bear? You begin to toy with the idea of drastic surgery. Americans are used to instant gratification, and you may be willing to
jump on the bandwagon of anything promising a quick fix.

The quality of life has deteriorated to the point that obese
people will take great risks to gamble with the reversal of their
obesity. If you are even contemplating such measures, please
check out the chapter on gastric bypass surgery.

At this crucial time in your life, you realize it's now or never. You are weary of struggling with this issue. You don't want
this terrible self-image and feeling of defeat. You realize that if
you don't solve this problem soon, your health will deteriorate
while your inferiority complex will grow. You don't want another child staring at you or pointing fingers or asking embarrassing questions about you or your classmates making fun of
you or your peers at work feeling sorry for you because you are
overweight. You hate your feelings of inadequacy and inferiority around people who are normal. You feel so inept. You've

tried and failed so many times. You are discouraged and hopeless. I'm here to give you hope!

It should be simple, and it is. My forty years of extreme dieting methods began with my teenage years. I have always believed that dieting should not be complicated. Food should not need to be measured or weighed or counted in grams or calories or carbs or have its glycemic index measured. That is unnatural to human behavior. Those things can be used as tools, but they shouldn't consume your time and energy for the duration of your life. I searched for a workable plan until I stumbled across a way of eating that was unbelievably simple, yet effectively removed all sugar cravings. The golden key to dieting success was always right under my nose. I didn't know that there was a way to stop sugar cravings. Sugar cravings are never satisfied. Eating processed sugar only magnifies the problem, while making you crave more food and more sweets. Processed sugar keeps your appetite in high gear, keeping you constantly hungry. That's why it's so difficult to control.

I enjoy studying the people in old photos and movies. In our local Dairy Queen, one wall is covered by an old black-and-white photo of hundreds of people waiting to get ice cream when a Dairy Queen opened decades ago. Did you ever notice how thin those people appear? You don't see the fat or obesity levels that are commonplace today. People ate differently then and were much more active—and it shows! Did you know that airlines, churches, and stadiums are making seats wider to accommodate our increasing bulk? One Japanese gentleman joked that they could seat forty thousand Japanese citizens in their stadium or twenty thousand Americans. This is not a laughing matter anymore. Why is this happening to people in all cultures who switch to our Western diet?

If you are a sugar addict, you will never eat chocolate and not want more. You can never finish off the last gallon of ice cream and not crave more. If potato chips are your thing, you can never eat one and not reach for the next. White-flour products such as breads, rolls, and bagels can also raise your insulin levels and increase your hunger. If you find that you can't stop at one bagel, one roll, or one slice of bread, then you need to stop, breathe, shift gears, and keep reading. Diets don't work if they don't crush the cravings. I have tried limiting my amount of sweets to only once a day or once a week, but the cravings overwhelmed me. Trying to eat just one chocolate chip cookie or one small scoop of ice cream is like trying to stop the waves from crashing on the beach. For a sugar addict, there is no such thing as one bite, one scoop, or one small serving of something sweet.

Just visually seeing leftover desserts would trigger my cravings, and I could think of nothing else until those cravings were satisfied—*now!* My intense addiction drove me to seek instant gratification by eating more sweets. Often, I would not even taste what I was eating after several bites. I would inhale, and the snack would be gone. An hour later, I would be craving sweets again. I would walk past the same spot to see if there was any left, and just like a drug addict, I would scarf up any crumbs remaining. During that time, I thought of little else except the possibility that there might be a leftover cookie or donut or brownie in the office kitchen. My mind would not give me rest until I jumped up and checked. By then, my taste buds and cravings would be in such a frenzy that if the cookies or donuts were depleted, I would raid the candy machine or make a trip to the cafeteria dessert counter.

If I had an appointment with the bank, I would specifically plan to spend my lunch hour at the ice cream shop next door. I'd decide before I got there whether I would order chocolate ice cream, chocolate chip cookies, or chocolate glazed donuts. Sometimes, I would order all three. After all, I reasoned, I only stopped by the bank once a month, so it was okay to treat myself. It's a wonder I didn't pass out from sugar-shock. There were many times when I literally made myself ill from the overconsumption of sweets.

If I had an evening class or event, I would leave early enough to stop by the frozen yogurt shop on the way and have a large container of chocolate frozen yogurt.

Isn't it ironic that when certain people are faced with lung cancer or heart disease, they immediately stop smoking or revolutionize their eating habits or reduce their stress by making drastic life changes? It's easy to ignore the warning signs until the situation becomes life threatening. I'm glad that same urgency happened to me.

It took several episodes of strange heart palpitations to turn me around dramatically. At age fifty-three, my heart did something unthinkable. Three different times in a one-week span, I found it difficult to breathe. My heart pumped erratically. The feeling passed in a few seconds, but each time the episode lasted longer, until the third time I struggled to breathe for what seemed like a minute. During each occurrence, it was very difficult to draw in enough oxygen and I felt myself struggling for life. Each of these episodes appeared within hours of eating a particularly large amount of sugar. The third episode lasted long enough and scared me to the point that I decided my eating patterns had to change immediately. I did not want to go through another episode and give myself a heart attack or stroke from poor eating habits. I did not want to put myself into an early grave out of stupidity. I knew enough about nutrition to understand that I was a sugar junkie and to solve this health issue I would need to go off my addiction "cold turkey." At this point, the thought of possible weight loss wasn't even the issue. What happened next, I never expected. Good things beyond my wildest dreams resulted in that life-changing decision. But first, I had to act upon that decision.

Since my teenage years, I've been all the way from 112 pounds (which lasted all of about three hours after an unhealthy crash diet) to 210 pounds several times, when I wasn't pregnant. Weighing 210 unnerved me so badly that I starved myself below 200 each time. Something about staying over 200 pounds was intolerable to me. There was no way I could ratio-nalize being that heavy, but we all have our tolerance levels. You might ask yourself, what number do you tolerate? Being over 150 pounds was also obese for me, but 200 pounds was easier to maintain.

During pregnancy, I gained sixty pounds because I was ravenously hungry and eating too many sugared foods, which triggered greater hunger and kept me in the vicious cycle of gaining and eating. I lost only fifteen pounds at the birth of my baby. That was depressing. At the time I was so inexperienced and so upset with all that weight gain that I barely ate. My baby was nursing nonstop, and I didn't know why. My older and more experienced sister asked me how much I was eat-ing. When I realized that I wasn't eating enough to nourish my baby, I went back to eating plenty but made wrong choices in foods.

Sometimes in earlier years I dieted down to a reasonable weight but attracted so much attention from the male species that it made me extremely uncomfortable. Even though I en-joyed being thinner, I didn't know how to maintain my weight. Moreover, I was way too shy and untrained in the social graces to know how to handle male attention adequately. To avoid social interaction that I found extremely stressful, I preferred to melt into the background instead. While heavier, I noticed that less positive male attention was directed toward me, so that didn't reinforce a better self-image either. By middle age, I de-veloped a much healthier perspective of self and strengthened my social interaction skills so that I could move past awkward issues. I would never choose to remain heavy now to avoid dealing with people. Heaviness is unhealthy and should not be used as an excuse to avoid social situations.

When the liquid protein diets were popular, I fasted for three days on that awful fluid but couldn't stand the taste, ex-perienced hunger constantly, and hated the lack of variety, so I quit. Thank God for that, because it was killing people. Their hearts stopped. I've tried the latest in diet pills, which either caused me to experience diarrhea, intestinal cramps, insomnia, or a racing heartbeat. Most diet pills caused such adverse side effects within twenty-four hours that I stopped their use immediately; of course, I was already poorer, as those items were always overpriced and could not be returned for refund. The other diet pills did absolutely nothing to help me lose weight either, but each time put hundreds of dollars in someone else's pocket. If pills or diet drinks affected my body negatively, I knew my health was more important than mere weight loss, so I would discontinue that product and move on to the next.

I've also tried the sweetened diet drinks, but those increased my hunger because of the high amounts of added sweeteners.

I've experienced the diets that came with already prepared and prepackaged food (I almost starved on those), any diet that seemed sensible, and others that made no sense at all. I've spent considerable amounts of money on diets and pills containing collagen and herbal or enzyme miracle cures that promised to solve all my weight problems but didn't work for me. My metabolism slowed to a crawl, and it became harder to lose weight. My body seemed to sense that it should go into starvation mode and store fat whenever I began a different style of eating. It got to the point where I could stay on a consistent low-calorie diet for weeks and actually gain weight while my energy level plummeted because I wasn't eating enough healthy food. I felt awful physically and was hungry constantly.

Once I fasted for twelve days with nothing to eat but water and vitamins. It takes willpower to accomplish something as crazy as that, so I didn't lack willpower. I lost over twenty pounds but gained it back in three days because my body's cells became so depleted for nourishment, they screamed for food. A year later I fasted again for nine days with nothing but water but lost only six pounds and added about ten pounds back in two days because my body rebelled. I had no strength during the fast because my metabolism jumped into starvation mode. It was conserving energy as it sensed that there was a serious famine going on again. My body demanded retribution for starvation, and my hunger was so great that after breaking each fast I ate everything in sight to make up for becoming malnourished.

I've tried counting calories, but my hunger always won eventually. I counted carbs. I counted fat grams. I carried little books in my purse to check the calorie, carb, and fat content of every item I was eating. It all seemed so futile, though I was building knowledge about what didn't work for me.

I've always achieved other goals. It frustrated me that I could not seem to control diet and proper weight. Food is a double-edged sword. Until you learn to choose the foods that will help your body operate efficiently, you will be unable to maintain. I needed food to survive but hadn't yet figured out that certain foods were causing my enormous cravings and larger appetite. Since dessert was one of my biggest enjoyments in life, I thought it would be impossible to give it up completely. Wrong! I was wrong to believe that sweets were actually one of my biggest comforts and wrong to think that they would be impossible to give up. Today, I don't even miss sweets. Through this book, I want to share that journey with you and help you reach your goals.

If you've been around for a few decades, you've probably noticed that Americans are becoming fatter. You may be appalled at yourself for being one of them. If you are more than a few decades old, you probably remember how few teenagers in your grade school or high school were fat. Our eating habits and the types of foods we are eating have changed drastically since 1950. Look around you today. The neighborhood is filled with fat babies, fat toddlers, fat children, fat teenagers, and fat adults. Almost two out of three adult Americans are considered overweight. Ours is the first generation to be bombarded with poor quality foods. Is your weakness sweets, alcohol, salty snacks, other junk food, or all of the above? It doesn't help that we have easy, unlimited access to these items today and barely have to lift a finger to stuff ourselves.

What food drives you to leave your warm, comfortable abode and burn gas at three dollars per gallon to get across town until you have the food in your hand and in your mouth before leaving the parking lot? What food is on your mind from the time you wake up until you collapse into bed exhausted at the end of the day? If you are thinking about that substance hours before the next meal and gravitate toward that same item every day, you have a food addiction. How can you get free of a food addiction? Is it possible to not be tempted by milk chocolate ice cream or bread rolls ever again? Yes, it is possible, but it will take your resolve from several days to two weeks to break that habit and become free of your addiction! Once you become addiction-free, you need to keep away from those temptations for at least two months, until you are firmly fixed in your new lifestyle habit. That way nothing on earth will ever move you to return to that hopelessness of getting nowhere anytime soon.

CHAPTER 2

Obesity Stalks the Earth

"My problem is sugar, not my willpower."

OBESITY IS BONDAGE. It's suffocating. It robs you of a quality life. It steals your happiness. You become a slave to your slowed-down, heavier body, which can often be attributed to an out-of-control food addiction to sugared products, chocolate, salty junk foods, or breads. Obesity is the road to poor health. Type two diabetes, heart disease, knee replacements, and numerous other surgeries await you. When you stay obese, you cannot avoid serious surgeries and health problems in your future. There is an easier way to get off this endless treadmill!

It was always frustrating that a small chocolate bar could seemingly turn into five pounds of weight gain overnight. Now chemists know that this has a lot to do with the way our body stores fat and what is causing too much of that fat storage in the obese individual: processed sugar.

Have you ever heard a normal-weight person say, "I forgot to eat"? That has never been a problem for those of us who live to eat, but now we know why. Sugar attacks our bodies by flipping the "on" switch to hunger.

Our body was not designed to live on refined sugar, no fiber, and processed foods devoid of minerals and vitamins. **When we glut our flesh with these non-foods, the appetite** (controlled by the brain center) will never be satisfied because it is not receiving what it needs to repair itself or function properly.

Hamster in the Wheel

How often have you felt like you couldn't escape this nightmare of fatness and overeating the wrong types of foods? Like the fat little hamster running forever on his wheel but never getting anywhere, that is exactly what we are doing when we continue to eat sweets or junk foods. We can't stop eating these types of food long enough to get off our wheel, look around, and find another purpose in life. Our own addiction to sugar or snack foods keeps us running (or waddling) in the same direction without end. Borderline insanity is expecting to get different results while doing the same things over and over. So let's get *sane*!

Sugar Is Making You Fat

For most obesity problems, sugar and other junk foods are the culprits standing between you and your ideal weight. If sugar is your trigger food to overeat, then sugar is making you fat. If you find that you overeat all snack foods (usually composed of processed sugars, white flours, or salty items), then you need to identify and make a list of foods that trigger you to excess. We used to believe that fat was the culprit, so everyone jumped on the no-fat diet bandwagon and gained weight! Since that time, the truth has surfaced about how crucial essential fats and oils are to properly functioning body chemistry (I will discuss these further in later chapters). You can and will gain weight if you overeat non-fat sugary foods or non-fat junk foods such as pretzels.

For most of us, the trigger food for overeating is sweets. For others, overeating can be exaggerated by any food that lacks nutrition or fiber but causes you to keep eating (such as pretzels, potato chips, or cheese crackers). One friend could not understand why she gained weight when all she snacked on between meals was an entire bag of non-fat pretzels every day. Non-fat snack products can cause you to overeat and therefore cause you to gain enormous amounts of fat. Had my friend chosen raw carrots instead of pretzels, she would not have gained weight because the fiber, vitamins, and minerals in those carrots would have filled and satisfied her appetite. **Beware of non-fat foods that keep you snacking all day long because they lack fiber and essential minerals and nutrients.** Therefore, these products are not satisfying and do not feed your body what it needs. Instead, they keep your metabolic system in a constant state of "hunger."

Cows gain weight quickly if fed a diet high in grain products. People who can't leave breads and pastas (which are made from grain) alone often have the same result.

Too many people fail at dieting because of a gulping or overeating mechanism that kicks in when they eat unhealthy substances that lack nutrients. You can end the sugar or junk food habit. Does giving up sugar or nutritionally starved snacks sound too much like deprivation? Actually, kicking the poor snack habit will set you free to really enjoy your life. Up to this point, you only thought you were enjoying life by burying your face in a swill of disease-causing, heart-stopping, processed-sugar-infested products. Once you become free of this addiction, you will realize how seducing its mere taste is. That's all the hold that sugar or snack foods have on you. An addiction to the sweet taste of processed sugars or the salty taste of pretzels or potato chips can never be satisfied as long as you continue to allow them into your body.

Just because you are addicted to sweets does not mean you are weak-willed. We're born to love a sweet taste.

Since my nemesis is sugar, processed sugars are the main focus in this book. The definition of nemesis from Webster's dictionary is "one that inflicts retribution or vengeance. An unbeatable rival. A source of harm or destruction." That pretty much sums up the problem that you are facing.

In a prehistoric world, finding sugar—mostly honey or wild berries—was a rare chance to stock up on calories along with plenty of nutrients and much needed fiber. But today, we live in a world where we're surrounded by endless chances to eat delicious, sugar-loaded foods—at malls, the office, the movies, gas stations, bookstores, and our own homes. Ironically, our inborn love of sugar is now a health liability, bringing more calories on board than we can burn in a day. However, we can break the addiction to sugar and stop the vicious eating cycle.

The first step in recognizing the scope of the problem is to define just how sugar crazy we are as a society. The average American eats from sixty to ninety pounds of sugar per year from high-fructose corn syrup, dextrose, invert sugar, fructose, barley malt, cane sugar, malt syrup, and all the other sugars that are added to and often hidden in processed food. **Unfortunately, there is not one shred of anything in processed sugar that will contribute to your good health.**

Most of those empty calories come from non-diet soft drinks, candy, sweet baked goods (such as cakes, cookies, and donuts), ice cream, and sweetened fruit drinks. At the top of the list are soft drinks. Gone are the days when our children drank milk at every meal. Refrigerators are filled with sugar-flavored, carbonated, color-dyed soft drinks that are wreaking havoc with our insulin levels, allergies, and overall health. They contribute one-third of the added sugar in our average United States diet, which is not surprising when you realize that one twenty-ounce bottle of Coke has **seventeen teaspoons of sugar**, making it the equivalent of liquid candy. Our children are developing asthma, ear infections, and type two diabetes at an unprecedented rate, and sugar-related health problems are increasing every year. A lethal dose of sugar is clogging our sensitive systems and **causing** many of our health problems.

If you think that sweetened fruit drinks are any better for

your health, they are not. These drinks contain mostly added sugar or sweeteners, colored dyes, and water, with a tiny pinch of real juice thrown in for flavor or to be able to print "real fruit juice" on the label. You would need a good chemist to find any real fruit juice in a fruit drink that is not labeled 100 percent fruit juice. The pretty labels showing lovely whole fruit in bright colors are meant to throw you off guard. After all, the more you pay for pretty sugar-flavored, colored water, the less it costs the manufacturer to make and the more money goes into their pockets. It's much cheaper to mix plain tap water with dye and flavorings than to pay the farmer to grow it, pick it, transport it to market, preserve it, strain it, and bottle it as 100 percent fruit juice.

If you remember that one teaspoon of sugar is four grams, you can generally figure out how much sugar is in today's processed foods. Processed foods do not grow naturally in nature. Oreo cookies aren't picked from a tree. Coca-Cola does not come from a fresh mountain stream gushing out brown-flavored, carbonated sugar water.

If you drink just one twenty-ounce Coke and eat ten Oreo cookies in one binge, you have already consumed over twenty teaspoons of sugar in one day. You are a ticking time bomb before type two diabetes and other horrible diseases control your body.

A coffee latte a day at over two hundred calories and eight teaspoons of sugar can increase your weight by one more pound every seventeen days unless you are burning it off in exercise.

If you consume only one-seventh of an Entenmann's Louisiana Crunch Cake, you will have devoured eleven teaspoons of sugar.

You may think you're doing yourself a favor by eating fruit-flavored yogurt, but don't be fooled. One eight-ounce Dannon vanilla yogurt contains over eight teaspoons of sugar.

I used to wonder how my mother could drink a glass of

plain buttermilk every day. Now I occasionally crave unsweetened plain yogurt. It's the only yogurt that doesn't have any processed sugar or artificial sweeteners. Sometimes I add real fruit for the extra punch of flavor.

If you are a sugar addict, just limiting yourself to one sweet treat per day is pushing you right over the edge into sugar dependency and constant cravings. That one small 1.69-ounce package of M&M's contains almost eight teaspoons of sugar.

One Hostess Low Fat Chocolate Cup Cake or a 1.6-ounce package of Reese's Peanut Butter Cups packs a walloping five teaspoons of sugar. Who among us has the willpower to stop at just one?

One twelve-ounce can of Mountain Dew is giving you an insulin rush of 11.5 teaspoons of sugar, while a twelve-ounce can of Seagram's Ginger Ale only contains nine teaspoons of sugar. Is it any wonder that our blood sugar levels are going berserk and type two diabetes is increasing?

If you can't leave ice cream alone, one pint of Haagen-Dazs Caramel Pecan ice cream contains about eight-and-a-half teaspoons of sugar, while one pint of Ben & Jerry's Chunky Monkey frozen yogurt contains the equivalent of ten teaspoons of sugar.

I used to drink Arizona Original Iced Tea, but a twenty-ounce container holds fifteen teaspoons of sugar. If you are tricked into believing that any drink with "fruit" in the name must be healthy for you, take a look at a twenty-ounce container of grape-flavored Fruitopia, which contains over nineteen teaspoons of sugar. Snapple Orangeade in the twenty-ounce size contains over fourteen teaspoons of sugar. This is enough sugar to put many diabetics into a coma, **and it is wreaking havoc in your body, even if you don't feel it yet.** It is only a matter of time before you will suffer from arthritis, and you may mistakenly attribute it to aging, when the real cause is sugar infestation in your body. You don't have to be obese for the effects of sugar to undermine your health. Many people notice a huge decrease in their aches and pains only days after deleting processed sugar from their eating patterns and filling that void with fresh fruits and vegetables.

Women seem to veer toward sugar because we are our own worst enemies, especially with our hormones peaking at different times during the month. We are always in a hurry to lose weight, so we cut out nutritious snacks and go too long between balanced meals. Then our blood sugar dives. After we grab a sugary snack to pick us back up, the sugar sets off hunger cravings that become impossible to ignore; we cause our own dieting nightmares.

Sugary foods are high-glycemic and are digested faster than other foods. The sugars release into the bloodstream and rapidly overload the system so that cells begin storing fat at an accelerated rate. That triggers a bigger insulin response in some people, **causing calories to be quickly stored** rather than kept available for quick energy. The result? We actually get hungrier sooner—and eat more. **Therefore, we gain weight rapidly**.

It isn't too difficult to see that eliminating sugar results in a slimmer body.

Giving up processed sugar takes commitment, and you'll probably feel irritable at first. Just remember the role that sugar plays in weight gain. Plus, here's some good news: once sweets are gone (and the cravings are out of your system), you will find to your amazement and disbelief that you no longer miss them. Some people reach that point in as little as five days, while others with severe sugar addiction take around two weeks to clean out their system. This was true in my case. Your taste preferences will change dramatically. It wasn't until I no longer craved sugar that I developed a taste for plain, unsweetened yogurt. Foods you used to avoid will suddenly become more appealing. You may even learn to like those stronger-flavored vegetables that you used to avoid. You will develop a taste for nutritionally vibrant foods—those that contribute to your health instead of destroying it.

You've got too much to live for to take your marching orders from a cupcake.

To determine if you are a sugar addict, you might ask yourself the following questions. If you have a problem with any one of these areas, it is undermining your ability to lose weight or keep it off permanently, and setting yourself up for health problems.

- Do you open a pack of cookies and eat them all in less time then it takes to inhale?

- Do you find yourself buying more than one pack of M&M's and eating every bag before you get home?

- If you don't have your chocolate every day, do you get irritable?

- Do you drive in rain, snow, sleet, or hail to get your sugar fix?

- Have you ever binged by eating the whole pack of cookies, the entire half gallon of mint chip ice cream, or six slices of lemon crème pie in one sitting? How about three slices?

- Do you get a slight headache without your chocolate fix every day?

- Is it hard to resist your favorite sweets? Do you burn extra gas or walk out of your way to get to your temptation? I used to take long walks and purposely select my route to pass an ice cream shop!

- Are you unable to eat just one bite of something sweet?

- Are you afraid or ashamed that if people knew how much sugar you really eat, they would be horrified? Do you eat sweets where no one sees you do it?

- Do you often tell yourself that you will not have sweets for a while, but then give in and feel guilty?

- Are you unable to say no to dessert every day after dinner?

Now truthfully admit whether or not you are a sugar addict. Repeat after me: "I am a sugar addict." Now how do you fix it?

When your blood sugar is out of balance from all the sweets you consume, you will feel tired too often, restless, and confused. You will have trouble remembering things or concentrating. You will become easily frustrated, find yourself more irritable than usual, and get angry unexpectedly. Does this sound like you or any of your children? What are they eating?

Calories Add Up

If you eat just one hundred calories a day over what you need, that's enough to make you gain ten pounds in one year. Many sugar addicts can easily consume over one thousand extra calories per day, so unless you are actively burning off that excess poundage with extreme amounts of intense exercise, you are quickly turning into the Goodyear blimp.

It only takes about 3,500 extra calories to gain a pound of fat. Two cans of soda contain about 500 calories and a one-ounce bag of chips about 150 calories. If that is a typical snack each day for you or your child, it adds up to a pound of fat in five or six days, unless you engage in thirty to forty-five minutes of daily vigorous activity to burn it off. One out of every six children and teenagers today is overweight. In the United States, 75 percent of our population is expected to be overweight by the end of 2007. This should be alarming to all of us. We should be beating the drums for a healthy-food revolution in this country!

Instead of depriving you or your child of food, keep only nutritious choices around, such as whole fruits and nuts. The fiber will help you fill up faster, and your hunger mechanism will naturally shut off. Find ways to get involved in fun and active exercise that will be enjoyable. An excessively heavy person will find it difficult to enjoy being active. It will be a long, slow process but well worth the journey. The key is to eat foods loaded with fiber, vitamins, minerals, and living enzymes so you won't feel hungry and to find enjoyable activities that are not food related.

Don't worry about the sugar in sauces, soups, or other non-sweet foods, or the natural sugar in raw fruit or milk. That kind of sugar comes packaged with lots of good-for-you nutrients—and that's not where your excess weight is coming from. How often have you binged on too many apples or bananas?

Lose Weight Now

Disability increases with excess weight. Back pain, knee surgery, and type two diabetes—conditions frequently tied to excess body weight—can knock you out of work and into a hospital. If you want an active life, you must manage your weight by controlling what goes into your mouth.

Obesity Health Consequences

As I neared the age of forty, I heard the terms "fat, female, and forty" associated with many of the chronic diseases.

You don't have to be female or forty to be obese and have an increased risk for physical ailments such as the following:

- High blood pressure, hypertension
- High blood cholesterol, dyslipidemia
- Type 2 (non-insulin-dependent) diabetes
- Insulin resistance, glucose intolerance
- Hyperinsulinemia
- Coronary heart disease

- Angina pectoris

- Congestive heart failure

- Stroke

- Gallstones

- Cholescystitis and cholelithiasis

- Gout

- Osteoarthritis

- Obstructive sleep apnea and respiratory problems

- Some type of cancers (such as endometrial, breast, prostate, and colon)

- Complications of pregnancy, such as gestational diabetes, gestational hypertension, preeclampsia, and complications in operative delivery (i.e., C-sections).

- Poor reproductive health (such as menstrual irregularities, infertility, and irregular ovulation)

- Bladder control problems (such as stress incontinence)

- Uric acid nephrolithiasis

- Psychological disorders (such as depression, eating disorders, distorted body image, and low self-esteem)

In our culture, we are surrounded by the obese while the rate of type two diabetes quickly climbs. When I was a teenager, I only knew one person who was diabetic. Today, diabetes is becoming as common as acne! We are turning into a sickly society, mostly caused by what we're eating.

Excess weight and obesity are partners with diabetes, high blood pressure, high cholesterol, asthma, arthritis, and poor health in general.

As body fat increases, the risk of all of the above conditions increase as well.

Thinking and learning abilities get worse with type two diabetes, also nicknamed "diabesity." Dementia increases dramatically with any of the following factors: smoking, any type of diabetes, hypertension, and high cholesterol (because of the clogging of arteries, capillaries and therefore, decreasing oxygen flow to the brain).

Your Knees Are Buckling

Body weight is a major contributor to knee problems. It used to be unheard of for twenty-year-olds to have knee surgery if they weren't injured in sports events. Now, knee surgery operations are commonplace in all ages of the obese. Every ten pounds of excess fat is equivalent to an extra sixty pounds of pressure on your knee area, and you feel it if you accidentally step off a curb or miss the bottom step. If you are one hundred pounds overweight, that's an extra six hundred pounds of pressure on your knees. Is it any wonder that your knees are buckling under the strain of holding you up? It's like a Clydesdale draft horse walking on Shetland pony knees.

Medical teams are increasingly reluctant to operate on the knees of the obese. It takes obese individuals much longer to recover, and they are at a higher risk for triggering other life-threatening situations. Follow-up surgery is often required. More hospitals are requiring the patients to lose weight first or go without knee surgery. **Sometimes these same patients find out that after they lose weight, they no longer need knee surgery!**

Easy Food Decreases Exercise

As technology has made it easier to mass-produce large quantities of nutritionally dead foods cheaply, obesity from overeating these chemical food substitutes has increased. We have designed foods with preservatives and packaging that have ridiculously long shelf lives. Unless moisture gets into the package, some of these products may stay fresh longer than us!

What's really scary is that we will eat those dead foods without thinking about the effect it may have on our health. We've developed the technology but not the common sense to deprive ourselves of things that tickle our taste buds. Our society has become so advanced that energy expenditure is no longer a given for weight control. As our calorie intake goes up, our energy expenditure, or exercise, goes down. The wonderful advances of technology don't merely free us from tiresome toil to produce and harvest our own food, they make it almost impossible for us to get a decent amount of calorie-burning exercise.

Fat Boosts Blood Pressure

Excess fat isn't just ugly; it works its way inside your kidneys and heart, compressing them and stopping their ability to control fluid flow through your body. **Cutting body fat helps take the pressure off your kidneys and arteries, which makes it less likely that you will have a heart attack or premature kidney failure.**

Type Two Diabetes

Type two diabetes is caused by high sugar levels in the blood. **It is not an inherited disease. It is a way of eating, and what you are eating disease.** You can get rid of this disease completely by removing from your diet substances that contain added processed sugar and extremely sweet fruits such as oranges, grapes, and bananas. If you have type two diabetes, ask your doctor for more details of which foods to avoid. You can also look up the glycemic index charts at www.glycemicindex. com, which lists foods with higher sugar content. You should avoid these foods if you have type two diabetes.

There's nothing to blame for this epidemic except the way we eat. Type two diabetes is a lifestyle disease from excess body fat—caused by too much TV, too little activity, and high-calorie junk food.

Type two diabetes is the failure of cells to absorb glucose, the sugar molecules that fuel muscles, nerves, and the brain. When sugar cannot enter the cells, it builds up in the blood, leading over time to devastating complications: heart attack, stroke, kidney failure, and nerve damage, even limb amputation and blindness. When muscle and nerve cells are deprived of glucose, they function more slowly, explaining why early type two diabetes may reveal itself as tiredness and irritability. Unfortunately, our poor diets can lead to blindness, amputations, heart attacks, and strokes. This is nothing to fool around with. We are beginning to see so much type two diabetes around us that we have lost our fear of its seriousness. Merely consuming healthier foods and increasing our activity levels can erase or greatly reduce the dangers of this disease.

Anticancer Ally

Being obese triggers hormones that spur explosive growth in abnormal cells and set the stage for tumors.

While risk of the most common adult leukemia is almost double in overweight women, endometrial cancer, colorectal cancer, and esophageal cancer are also many times higher in the obese.

Drop Pounds before Pregnancy

If you are obese, your odds of having a successful pregnancy are low and your risk of miscarriage is considerably higher than your healthy-weight counterparts.

Obesity causes hormonal imbalances that make it harder to conceive and carry to term.

Take a Load Off Your Heart

The risk of a ballooning heart wall and related irregular beats increases significantly in obese people. Obesity may cause the heart's upper left chamber, the atrium, to stretch out and develop a too-rapid beat that's out of sync with the rest of the heart. This raises stroke risk significantly.

Obesity Ages You

People who are overweight are aging faster than their years. **Those extra pounds actually speed up the aging of the heart, arteries, brain, and other organs.** They also encourage the growth of breast tumors and prostate cancer. To add insult to injury, lugging around those extra pounds zaps your energy, making you feel tired and fatigued. All that weight also stresses out your joints and ligaments as they hold up all that poundage. That's why so many of the obese have hip or knee replacement surgery.

Sleep Apnea

If you have this disorder, you may experience many brief yet potentially life-threatening interruptions in your breathing while you sleep. Loud snoring, excessive daytime tiredness, and early-morning headaches are signs of apnea. Being overweight puts you at increased risk. Early treatment is vital because apnea is associated with irregular heartbeats, high blood pressure, heart attack, and stroke.

At two hundred pounds I could barely stay awake driving six miles to work. My daughter worried about me because I would stop breathing briefly many times during the night. Those scary symptoms have now disappeared.

Skip Dessert or Lose Your Mind

Obesity has been linked with memory and thinking problems. We have ceased to feed our brains foods that contain living enzymes to keep us functioning at peak level; instead we are feeding our fat.

Fat Is Actually a Living Organ

We used to believe that fat was just stored in our bodies and sat there as a result of too much chocolate or donuts, but it has recently been confirmed that **fat is actually a living organ that**

controls appetite, size, energy, fertility, how quickly we age, and our disease risk. In thinner people, fat has been found to curb appetite in a positive manner, boost metabolism, and work with other health-promoting hormones. This is why it is so important to eat nature-created fats and oils in your foods, such as the oil that comes from olives, fish, or nuts. Unfortunately, the extra store of fat in heavy people pumps out more chemicals that dull insulin sensitivity and promote inflammation, both of which raise the risk of chronic diseases such as cancer, type two diabetes, and heart disease, and interfere with the body's natural hunger signals. The best way to improve your health is to exercise more and refrain from junk foods.

Fatty Livers

NASH, or nonalcoholic steatohepatitis, is a deadly disease that is the single most common cause of abnormal liver function. It causes the same kind of liver damage as alcoholism. Currently, there is no effective treatment except liver transplantation in advanced cases. **What is very distressing is that this malfunction is now being found in children with fatty liver problems.**

This disease is caused when you consistently take in more calories than you burn off, and some of your fat is deposited in the liver, which becomes enlarged and fatty. Eventually, this fattiness leads to scarring (cirrhosis) and loss of functional liver tissue. The end result is liver failure.

Supersize

Just hours after you've eaten a typical fast-food lunch such as a mega-burger and a giant soda, fat globules start to obstruct your blood vessels. Continued consumption of these unhealthy meals can lead to heart problems, obesity, and type two diabetes.

The sooner you begin to wean yourself off unhealthy

foods, the quicker your health will stop deteriorating and your weight will stop increasing.

If you're a woman, you are now much more likely to die of fat-related conditions than you are to die of breast cancer (which also increases with large doses of sweets).

When you eat sweets, your insulin levels spike. High insulin levels increase your risk of breast cancer.

Overweight and on the Pill

The pill has been found to be less effective in preventing pregnancy in those who are obese.

Heart Disease and High Insulin

High insulin levels boost your blood fats, or triglycerides, and make it easier to get blood clots. Blood clots lead to heart attacks.

Carbs and Cancer

Carbohydrates don't cause cancer, but foods that quickly raise blood sugar levels—such as sugary products—increase the risk of colorectal cancer.

Santa Is Gaining Weight

Santa doesn't need the cookies anymore. Santa no longer even needs to add a pillow to appear fat. In the 1950s, huge sizes in clothing were unheard of, except for that rare, hard-to-size individual. Now there are a few shops that cater to extremely large sizes but they are difficult to find and rarely offer a wide selection of styles.

Asthma and Obesity

As weight goes up, asthma increases. Obesity is considered a risk factor for asthma, but **it's possible that the symptoms of wheezing and shortness of breath may be nothing more than signs of weight-stressed lungs.** Carrying lots of extra weight stresses breathing muscles, making them work harder and less effectively. The result: restricted airflow in the lungs, which produces asthma-like symptoms. It's entirely possible that you may not have allergies such as those associated with asthma, but rather your weight gain is short-changing your lungs' breathing capacity.

Breast Milk and Baby Health

When you're overweight, you produce less of the hormone prolactin, which is necessary for the production of adequate breast milk.

What's so good about breast milk? Breast milk has less sugar and fat and fewer calories than formula. Moreover, nursing takes more time and work than bottle-feeding, so breastfed babies are less likely to overeat and become overweight—a well-established risk for heart disease and Type two diabetes.

Formula-fed babies have increased chronic illnesses, such as earaches, infections, and asthma.

The lack of nutrition in poor-quality carbs has been linked to birth defects. Mothers who don't eat proper amounts of fruits, vegetables, dairy products, lean meats, and vegetables will have more miscarriages, babies with low birth weights, and babies that spend more time at the doctor's office or in the hospital. What the mother is eating will be passed to the child in the womb, just as her poor eating habits will later be passed to her growing children who follow her example.

Lower Your Cholesterol Naturally

High cholesterol can be lowered without medication merely by cutting down all animal products to a maximum of three servings per week. Changing your diet doesn't cause the severe side effects that high-cholesterol medications will bring. To lower your cholesterol naturally, cut all cheese, dairy products, meat, and fish to no more than three servings per week.

Increase your vegetable, nut, and fruit consumption. Stop eating all man-made margarines, and shift to olive oil.

If you want to know more, order nutritionist expert Ted Broer's books, DVDs, or CDs at www.healthmasters.com.

Cataracts and Weight

Keeping your weight in check protects your eyes. Fat people develop cataracts at a much earlier age than their lean counterparts. It only makes sense that what you are eating is affecting your sight.

Your Weight Ages Your Heart

Obese people have abnormal arteries that have lost their natural "stretchiness," setting the stage for atherosclerosis and eventually heart attacks and strokes.

Obesity Is Spreading

The obesity epidemic in the United States remains a major public health concern; the current obesity rate shows no signs of decline because our eating habits are getting worse. More U.S. adults are overweight than are normal or thin, and almost one out of six children is too heavy. These numbers are increasing each year.

America is getting fatter, and that includes children and babies. Parents are allowing their children to consume far too many sugary products. Babies are fed sweetened formulas and sweetened baby foods. We are contributing to their obesity and future health problems from the first moments of life. We only need to look around to see that we have lost our common sense. Fat kids and fat adults die younger because fat is infiltrating our organs and clogging our systems so that bodies cannot function properly.

We can easily reverse the trend by removing harmful foods from our homes and replacing these foods with healthy fruits and vegetables, lean meats, low-fat milk, and whole-grain products.

The world's populations are becoming fatter as income increases and more inhabitants leave rural areas and head for the cities. As the population fattens up, incidents of type two diabetes and high blood pressure also rise. Unfortunately, other countries seem to be adopting our Western diet of unhealthy foods and the diseases that follow.

Milk and Bones

Children are breaking more bones today than they were fifty years ago. It's estimated that today's children are drinking minimal amounts of milk and not getting enough calcium from other foods, while at the same time being less active. Sunshine is also important for the proper development of strong bones. Children who stay inside their homes day after day watching television or playing computer games are headed for softer bone density. Activity, sunshine, and calcium in healthy foods increase bone density.

Fat Kids

The percentage of overweight and obese children has been rising at an alarming rate. This causes depression and low self-esteem.

Obese children have a tougher time fitting in with other children. They are often teased, harassed, and embarrassed because of their excess poundage. Do your children a favor and encourage them as much as you can by removing harmful foods from your home and providing nourishing foods for their growing bodies. Give them plenty of foods to snack on, but make it products like apple slices and cheese. Wean them off sugar. Don't drink soda and expect them to drink milk. Don't eat cookies and expect them to adhere to a stricter way of eating. When you demonstrate good eating habits without obsessing over every calorie, children develop healthy attitudes toward food. Moms who don't count calories and don't worry about every little thing they eat have kids who are thinner and happier.

Each year doctors are seeing more children in their offices with obesity problems and major health issues associated with eating junk foods and getting little or no exercise.

It's not a coincidence that the same decades that brought us cable TV, home computers, the proliferation of fast-food restaurants, and huge portion sizes have also contributed to obesity. Additionally, many schools no longer offer recess or physical education, school lunches are high in fat and sugar, and there are vending machines in the hallways without healthy choices. We need to get the junk foods out of school lunchrooms and vending machines to keep our kids healthy.

Fitness = Smarts

Children and adults who are physically fit score higher on academic tests and have much better memories, reaction times, and problem-solving skills.

Set a Good Example

Parents need to eat the foods that they wish their children would eat. Children learn by emulating their parents' habits, and what you eat is your habit. If you never eat fruits or vegetables, then your children will not develop a taste for those foods. By eating fruits and vegetables, parents start a lifetime of cancer-fighting food habits without having to say a word. Hang in there. Keep offering fruits and vegetables that aren't immediate hits. It often takes many trials before kids accept a new food. Try fruit salads or real fruit shakes created in your blender and sweetened with 100 percent apple or grape juice.

Hyper Kids

If your child just can't sit still, there's a good chance the hyperactivity may be caused by artificial colorings and some common preservatives.

To see if tweaking your kids' diet could be the answer to their bouncing-off-the-walls dilemma or constant colds, try steering clear of artificially colored foods. Products like cheese puffs, bright yellow cheeses, and colored drinks often contain a combination of colored dyes that have been linked to hyperactivity in young children. Packaged macaroni and cheese, cheese snacks, and packaged popcorn with bright yellow dye are all culprits. Check the ingredient labels. They can be hidden in the most unlikely foods. Some types of red and blue dyes in drinks, children's vitamins, and dish soap have been linked to severe allergic reactions. Drinks and milk are not supposed to be blue, red, or bright yellow. Manufacturers, in their quest to sell more to an unsuspecting public, have thrown aside concern over public health for greed.

MSG (monosodium glutamate) is also highly toxic to certain adults and children and has been found in many children's products, from soup to crackers.

Our Western Diet in Far-Flung Places

The absence of refined carbohydrates protect against twentieth-century illnesses. Natives in other countries who have not been introduced to refined carbs or processed sugars do not suffer from high blood pressure, heart attacks, or the cancers so commonly seen in our western culture. As soon as our refined foods become the common diet of new industrial societies, these diseases begin to emerge.

The Pima Indians of Arizona have such a high rate of kidney failure from type two diabetes that their reservation has its own dialysis center.

In Saudi Arabia, type two diabetes and associated heart disease have emerged within a short generation after refined carbohydrates and a more Westernized diet became the norm.

By restricting simple carbohydrates, heart patients almost

always report improvement in symptoms and are able to reduce or stop medications for heart disease, high blood pressure, and/or type two diabetes.

When we eat a lot of desserts, bread, pasta, rice, and other highly processed starches and sugars, our ability to utilize insulin becomes impaired. We become insulin-resistant and glucose-intolerant. We put out excessive amounts of insulin, which in turn creates diabetes, hypertension, and atherosclerosis.

If you eat a high-carb diet, you're going to have a lot of leftover glucose in your blood, which your insulin promptly converts to fat. You get fatter, and you also feel tired all the time, partly because your cells aren't getting the fuel they need, and partly because the excess insulin drives your blood sugar levels below the optimal range. Your body can't convert all that excess sugar into fat fast enough to keep it from circulating in your bloodstream. **Excess sugar in the blood is very damaging. Your heart, blood vessels, kidneys, eyes, and nerves are particularly vulnerable.**

Even thin people are not safe from excess sugar in the blood. The mere process of growing older means that your cells are becoming somewhat resistant to glucose. A diet of highly refined carbohydrates ages you even more.

Large Waistline

If you tend to carry your weight around your waist and upper body, your risk for heart disease, high cholesterol, high blood pressure, and type two diabetes skyrockets. **Current guidelines define "high risk" as a waist that's greater than thirty-five inches for women or forty inches for men.**

My waistline did not fall below thirty-five inches until I dropped to 140 pounds. I heaved another sigh of relief at passing to the "safe" side of yet another red-letter danger point.

Office Discrimination

I don't care how fair you believe that you are or an employer says they are. As much as we pass laws to avoid discrimination against any difference in us, fat is considered less than beautiful in this culture and you are being discriminated against for that reason. Fat kids are mistreated at school, and fat adults are discriminated against whether or not it is intentional. Too much fat is disabling and unhealthy. It's costing companies their bottom line in rising health-care costs.

An obese person looks out of control and unhealthy. Obesity costs companies zillions of dollars in lost revenues, not only from higher insurance premiums for our sickening generation, but because fat people use extra sick time and make more doctors' appointments for back troubles, aching knees, high blood pressure, type two diabetes, and so on. Along with smokers, the obese generally use more prescription drugs and take more days off for sickness.

Articles are now appearing in well-heeled publications about the expenses of obesity to the employer and how certain companies are fighting back with higher premiums for their obese employees. This brings up another issue of assigning someone in the company to eyeball every employee and arbitrarily pick who they believe is obese to charge them higher premiums or to just charge the individuals who are actually driving up the premiums. Another way is to average out the higher costs and make every employee pay higher premiums, or dismiss those employees who are driving up costs for everyone else. It's a catch-22 as corporations are trying to squeeze out profits when medical costs are soaring.

Two Hundred Pounds of Trouble

My diet diary, begun in my teens, mentioned some of the obesity-driven health problems at two hundred pounds by age fifty-three.

- Numerous yearly colds, coughs, and voice loss

- Resting heart rate average of ninety beats per minute

- Knees ache.

- Wear size XXL or size 20–22W clothing

- Exhausted after climbing a flight of stairs

- Gasping for air with almost no exertion at odd moments

- Severe heartburn daily

- Throat closes suddenly while I'm awake and I gasp for air

- Sleep apnea with excessive snoring, and extreme sleepiness all day

- Driving over two miles is dangerous because I can barely keep my eyes open

- Frequent cramps occur in my toes, feet, or calves while driving or sleeping

- Hands hurt when opening a jar or removing a gas cap

- Legs ache after sleeping a few hours, compelling me to rise and walk for thirty minutes to relieve the pain, contributing to further sleep deprivation

- Need to visit chiropractor at least twice a month because of an old back injury

- If on my feet too long during the day, my legs ache all night

- While chewing I accidentally bite the inside of my cheeks because they are so fat

- Thighs and knees rub together

- I have three chins, one natural and the other two made of fat rolls

- Snow boots do not fit over my calves

- Clothes don't fit right

- Difficult to bend to put on shoes and socks or trim toenails

- Large fat bags hang from my belly, side hips, and lower back under the ribs

- Upper arms sag with fat

- Inner thighs slap together

- Hands hit my hips as I walk unless I hold them out away from my body

- Clothes are shapeless, matronly, and square looking

- Navel is bottomless

- Drive with my abdomen against the steering wheel (I'm vertically challenged, and my feet don't reach the foot pedals unless the seat is far forward.)

- Difficult to roll over or get up from the floor at this weight

- Sometimes fall over when I squat because I'm unbalanced from this weight

- Even my nose is storing fat

- Feel aged from poor nutrition and weight

- Feel constant embarrassment, guilt, condemnation, and shame

- People treat me differently because I'm fat; they are less courteous or caring

- Tired all the time

- Measurements are 47-47-50—similar to the shape of a blimp!

I encourage you to be totally honest with yourself and make your own list. Information is power. Power motivates you to take action. As I began losing weight, I scratched notes next to my list about the positive changes happening to me. Removing sugar from your diet will result in immediate changes. In only a few days of sugar abstinence, you will notice aches and pains disappearing.

You can read the statistics or problems facing the obese in almost every magazine and newspaper sold in the United States because it is our new national epidemic. Obesity hinders everything from prostate cancer screening to infertility.

Fat is health crippling and depressing. In our culture, fat dripping from every pore is not considered beautiful, even though more of us as adults are fat in this new millennium than of normal weight. Nevertheless, anyone not fitting into our cultural image of beauty is unfortunately considered "less acceptable."

Have you ever noticed that our favorite actresses are never heavy? God forbid that one of them should be human and gain a few pounds. Fat-bashing is the heavyweight sport of our media, and they are especially merciless with famous females. You rarely see the media making sport of the male actors that balloon outward. Only the female actresses are put through this torture. Our actresses and heroines must be beyond reproach, perfect, and flawless, but according to whose standards? Can we expect less of ourselves? Don't we notice our friends or children when they gain weight? Have we ever envied and admired the lone individual who lost all the weight, changed her lifestyle, made it off the fat roller coaster, and never went back, like Oprah? She fought the good fight, and she is keeping it off! We love a winner.

Before age twenty, I was rejected from joining a church choir and from admittance to a private college because of prejudice regarding my unacceptable weight. I was told flat out that these were the reasons that I was not accepted for either. Even though it hurt to be told that I wasn't good enough for their acceptance standards, I believed if they were that narrow minded, I would not have enjoyed being involved with them anyway. Unfortunately, my outer appearance made my flaw evident to the entire world, whereas other folks who might be hiding heinous personality traits could enter those same hallowed grounds without repercussion.

Olympian athletes are not heavy. These are the best of the best, the top of the line, and the cream of the crop. They devote hours each day to their sport, practicing, competing, and bending their bodies into impossible routines. They carefully monitor their food intake because they are driven by a common goal. They spend hours each day exercising to perfect their sport. They love to compete. They want to be the fastest, the strongest, the most graceful, and the ones who don't stumble in front of a worldwide audience. We cheer them on because we admire their tenacity and their perseverance. We love perfection. No one remembers a loser. Can we push ourselves to get that involved with our own health?

My dad used to tell me that I was "two ax handles wide." Though it bothered me immensely and hurt my feelings, I knew there was also truth in what he was saying. Later, when he suffered from dementia and was even less inhibited, he would look at my widening figure and ask "aren't you ashamed of yourself?" I never held it against him because his mind was slipping, but there was also that segment of truth that couldn't be ignored and the emotional hurt that went with it.

Yes, I was ashamed of getting fat, but at that time in my life, I hadn't yet figured out how to lose the weight and keep it off. I continued to exercise consistently, which prevented much weight gain, but I also allowed too many unhealthy foods into my system that triggered hunger and uncontrollable cravings. I believed that I would one day learn to control the amount of sweets that I put into my mouth. Instead, sugar controlled me so that I felt betrayed by my own inability to stop the cravings, and I was baffled by my predicament.

Where I used to eat an entire package of Oreo cookies within minutes, now I am completely satisfied for hours with a slice of cheese or one whole raw fruit. In my obese life, I would demolish a half gallon of milk chocolate ice cream in one sitting or an entire batter of chocolate chip cookie dough and then mix up another batch so that there would be enough for cookies. If I bought large bags of chocolate candy for the trick-or-treaters, I would eat all the chocolate bars and have to repurchase. After doing that several years in a row, it dawned on me to switch to candies I didn't like and, therefore, had no desire to eat. In eating these sugary foods, it was difficult to stop after the first bite. My addiction took over, and I could not really even taste the food. However, it was compulsive behavior to keep eating until it was gone. I kept stuffing myself until I could eat no more—the sign of a true addictive response.

After high school, I took a summer job as a waitress. I devoured all the leftover desserts untouched by the customers. It was at that point in my life, while still a teenager, that I made a life choice to never work in the food industry again because of my uncontrollable inclinations toward sweets. I noticed that most of the waitresses were heavy. Serving food all day made it too tempting to overeat. Other workers in the food industry told me that they tired of the candy or ice cream after a few weeks, but I never did. If I had not made that life choice while very young, I believe I would have become much heavier earlier in life. I should mention that I lived in a rural community and was also biking twelve miles to that restaurant and twelve miles home every evening, so the weight did not increase as quickly as it could have; and I was in excellent physical condition. Those were years when the world was much safer, and parents didn't fear for their daughter's safety biking or walking to work alone in rural America.

Even though I enjoyed making pies, cakes, and cookies, I stopped making those desserts decades ago to add some control to my situation. I limited my sweets to places "away from home."

I grew up in the boonies of the upper Midwest, where towns were few and far between and farms were off the beaten path. Since I didn't make enough wages as a waitress to help my parents support a second car, the only method of transportation available to me was biking or hiking. The nearest town that offered work was twelve miles away. After a few months of this hectic life and enduring another northern winter, I followed the hoards of graduating high school seniors who chose to leave home and head for the big city.

I found a desk job within days, but my eating patterns deteriorated somewhat with my newfound independence. Though I continued to take long walks in the California sunshine, my daily activities no longer required the physical demands I was accustomed to on the farm, so the weight gain advanced rapidly. Over the next thirty-some years, I rode that tidal wave of gain and loss while trying to get a handle on my unusual craving for sweets.

While my daughter was growing, I made the choice not to keep desserts in the house except for those rare times during major holidays. She grew up on fruits, vegetables, and protein dishes and actually craved spinach for a time while she was in high school. She'd come home from school and prepare herself some steamed spinach, which was most unusual sustenance for a teenager. We never purchased high-sugared cereals. If you are allowing your children to eat that stuff for breakfast every day, you may want to reconsider. Your children will get more sugar in one serving of sugared breakfast cereal (over ten teaspoons) than what the FDA recommends for an entire day per adult. Remember, the FDA only sets numbers according to what they believe won't kill you. Your body can get along just fine without any processed sugar.

Plain Cheerios and Raisin Bran were the breakfast cereals of choice available to my daughter, simply because they contained much lower amounts of sugar than most kids' cereals. We often cooked scrambled eggs for breakfast on the weekends or ate a large brunch at the local restaurant. My daughter didn't particularly like milk once she started school, but she would drink large amounts of 100 percent pure orange juice daily, so I never worried about her not getting enough calcium or vitamin C.

When my child was young, I had to plead with the elderly lady next door to stop handing my daughter candy every time she walked past. People may have the best of intentions, but they encourage the worst of habits.

We have to constantly guard against neighbors who like to feed all the neighborhood children sweets. Of course, it destroys their appetite for meals, and attributes to their crankiness and inability to fall asleep at a decent hour, let alone the damage it does to their growing bodies. A child needs to have foods that count toward nourishing growth and developing cells. To eat dead and plastic foods on a daily basis deteriorates and erodes health and development.

Weight Size and Bone Framing

To determine what weight might be best for you, review the website at Metropolitan Life www.halls.md/ideal-weight/met. htm.

To ascertain whether you have a small, medium, or large frame, check out your wrist size *in relation to other people of the same sex of average weight.* If most wrists are much larger than yours, you probably have small framing. Generally and most unfortunately, people with petite framing break bones easily. We once lived next to a teenage boy who had a small bone frame but whose sole pleasure in life was riding his skateboard. After his third broken bone in less than a year, his parents banned the skateboard from his list of entertainment activities.

I consider my bone framing medium because I don't have tiny wrists, but then again, I don't have as wide a wrist size as some other women of normal weight.

Make a game out of it the next time you're with a group of women at a meal or baby shower. Ask them all to hold out their wrists and tell you what their framing size is. It will certainly create a lively discussion and allow you to compare wrist sizes.

Dietary Guidelines to Get America Fit

The obesity epidemic in the United States has prompted our government to issue new dietary guidelines to get us back on the path to better health. These guidelines focus on eating less to reduce calorie intake and on increasing physical activity. Our government says we need to eat more fruits, vegetables, and whole grains. It now recommends a daily intake of two cups of fruit and two and one-half cups of vegetables, with at least three ounces of whole-grain products daily. The new food chart also recommends consuming three cups of low-fat or fat-free milk daily.

Exercise is also a key component to getting fit. Our government recommends sixty minutes of moderate to vigorous activity daily to maintain body weight and prevent weight gain. If people do what is good for them, it will help prevent heart disease, some cancers, and type two diabetes.

Our government goes to a lot of expense to make guidelines that are meant to be helpful (and which we as citizens pay for), but unless each individual takes responsibility for his or her own actions regarding what is put in the mouth and whether exercise is part of the daily routine, tax dollars spent on this study are futile. There will always be junk-food manufacturers who don't care if what they produce is healthy for the populace, and there will always be plenty of unhealthy foods around for each individual to choose to avoid. We must learn to maneuver ourselves responsibly through the minefields of empty calories.

Body Fat Index

Being obese is not just body weight but also the percentage of body fat. One may be of normal weight or underweight but still have excessive body fat due to lack of muscle mass. Inversely, someone who is overweight by a normal index but has low body fat is not considered obese (again because of muscle mass).

Once I learned about the body fat index, I estimated myself somewhere near the 40 percent body fat range at 210 pounds. An "allowable" BFI (body fat index) for my age of fifty-five to fifty-nine is around 27 percent. That's more fat than is necessary. I've found that I can hold the line at a lower percentage by keeping processed sugar and unhealthy snack foods out of my life.

Use the Body Fat Index at www.nicemuscle.com/body-fat-index.htm to determine whether you are normal or obese. Estimate your body fat index:

(1) Multiply your weight in pounds by 703. In my case, 130 pounds × 703 = 91,390

(2) Multiply your height in inches by itself. In my case, 62″ × 62″ = 3844″

(3) Then divide the answer in (1) by the answer in (2). In my case, 91,390 ÷ 3844 = 23.8%. Not bad considering my age! Remember, this is not entirely accurate because there is no way a math calculation can actually measure your body fat. It may appear that you have a high level of body fat, when in reality you might be very muscular. In addition, this calculation cannot take into consideration your frame size, but it will give you a rough estimate for general purposes. Either way, don't get too hung up on these figures.

Getting healthy has to become more important to you than remaining fat. When my health became the issue and I realized that I could die immediately of a heart attack or stroke if I kept sugar-binging, it was over in a heartbeat. I chose the road of health and longevity to be around for my grandchildren. Overnight I chose a healthier lifestyle and decided I would not put any obvious processed sugar into my mouth for at least one month. Fear drove me to do the right thing. That was my road to recovery. I did not want to die from my own dysfunctional poor eating habits and leave my grandchildren because of foolish eating choices. After that first month passed, I realized it was so much easier to live without sugar than to try and control the amount. Without sugar in my life, I didn't have to struggle with a weight problem or the cravings of the sugar addiction. **It is easier to eat no sugar at all than to try and restrain myself once I've had the first taste.** Once the sugar is out of your system, you will no longer have to fight against the sweet cravings that make you want to overeat.

Let me not pass from this Earth until I have won the battle and made better choices so that my children and grandchildren will also know how to choose that road by example. I don't want them to remember me as the grandmother who was too tired to play with them or the fat grandma who died with a half gallon of ice cream clutched in her hand, or the person who gave them unhealthy habits.

You have to clear the stumbling blocks out of your path. Get every addictive food out of your house, car, and office drawers while you are clearing your body of this addiction. Don't go near the dessert table at your friend's wedding. Eat plenty of protein and vegetables before you attend any party, or don't go at all during the time you are getting cravings out of your system. Avoid the lunchroom at work or any area where there will be leftover donuts, cookies, or items you can't resist. What have you got to lose except something that is not healthy for you anyway?

You only have to avoid these areas for the period of time it takes to cleanse your body from cravings (approximately one to two weeks) and to make it a lifestyle habit (about two months). After the cravings are gone, it won't bother you to walk past leftover chocolate chip cookies or donuts as long as you don't reach for one from habit. You will have the power to resist them because your cravings won't be driving your appetite wild. Even today, years after beginning this lifestyle of eating, I open and close the refrigerator door looking for something to eat from years of habit, not from hunger. I keep my unsweetened green tea pitcher filled and will pause long enough to enjoy a glass. Then I move out of the kitchen and into living life.

It was so satisfying these past several years to not gain an extra five pounds from Halloween through New Years. Our office is flooded with desserts from well-meaning distributors and co-workers who just enjoy sharing samples of their holiday baking. I was not tempted to eat a single bite and left all that forbidden food untouched. At the end of the holidays, the rest of the crowd were confirming their New Year's resolutions to lose all the weight gained, while I enjoyed eating whatever I wanted of healthier foods and had no weight to lose. I especially appreciated those distributors who brought in baskets loaded with fruit, nuts, or cheeses.

Is Your Doctor the Best Source for Weight Loss?

Most doctors have not been trained to deal with all the various food addictions or the best way to encourage you to lose weight. Doctors in the American Medical Association usually have not taken a single course in basic nutrition. If you find a thin doctor who has never experienced weight issues, that doctor may be less than sympathetic to your problem. Many doctors themselves are severely overweight and don't have the patience or the time to deal with a "lifestyle" problem. If you are a sugar addict and your doctor is giving you a diet that allows you to eat simple carbohydrates of any kind (processed sugars), you will probably not lose weight and keep it off because any clump of sugar entering your body will cause a chain reaction of overeating.

Specialists in weight reduction have more experience and knowledge of your particular type of problem and may be able to encourage you, but the average individual probably cannot afford this luxury. You need to develop lifestyle habits for good health. Take responsibility for your own health. Only you know the deepest secrets of what you put into your mouth and what you eat in the isolated places of your car, bathroom, or where you stop on your way to and from the office. Only you know the location of every ice cream shop in your city. Most Americans are so addicted to their habits that they could not lose weight on the advice of anyone, unless they understand why they overeat in the first place, such as overeating from a sugar addiction.

CHAPTER 3

The Big Deal about Healthy Foods

"Health is my greatest wealth."

ALL CALORIES ARE NOT created equal. I cannot stress this enough. Again for emphasis: all calories are not created equal. If all you consumed in January was two thousand calories per day in desserts and you decided to completely change your diet in February to two thousand calories of green vegetables and lean meat, you would gain weight in January and lose weight in February. Processed sugar triggers your storage cells to store fat. String beans and lean meats trigger your cells to burn fat to release more energy.

Many Americans are eating plastic foods that haven't one shred of cell-building material in them. We've gotten away from nutrients in real food to eating manmade substitutes of various chemical sugars and strangely altered, chemically laced fats that have never seen an olive tree or an ear of corn. We've left behind the healthful benefits of honey and molasses and turned instead to highly refined sugars devoid of any nutrition, which creates havoc in our bodies' cells. We are eating prepackaged, highly processed, nutrient-depleted "foods" (I use that term loosely). Terrible diseases result, which are increasing at rates unprecedented in our history. Type Two diabetes, which used to be almost unheard of in our society or among children, is now commonplace. We have forgotten the dangers. You can get your leg amputated or go blind with diabetes of any kind. Your life expectancy is shortened. This is a deadly serious illness. Where extreme obesity used to be rare, it is now suffocating our society. **We are waddling across the pages of history as the most overfed and undernourished peoples of our planet.** We are literally stuffing ourselves to death. When citizens of other nations travel to our shores for the first time, their shocked initial reaction is "Americans are so fat!" Our average pampered pet gets better nutrition, but pets are also commonly overweight and under exercised in our culture.

Healthy foods feed your body nutritionally. Without nutrition providing adequate nourishment to your cells, you are sabotaging your own ability to lose weight because of constant hunger that drives you to excessive eating. Every gram of sugar you eat takes away calories of actual living foods that would nourish you.

Proper nutrition adds the sparkle to your eyes, sheen to your skin, luster to your hair, and moisture to your fingernails. Your body is constantly repairing and rebuilding itself, but only if it receives the proper nutrients from what you are eating. It needs protein, enzymes, vitamins, and minerals to function properly. Without adequate nutrition, disease knocks on your door. Much of the mental depression today is caused by a diet totally lacking in nutrition. Just gulping vitamin pills daily is not going to help if you are glutting yourself with the wrong substances. Most of today's highly processed fast foods or prepackaged snacks and sweets are nutritionally devoid of life-giving substances. You'd be better off eating a handful of dirt and would probably get better nutrition from the minerals (along with a few nasty parasites).

If food companies have to add vitamins and minerals to foods, that means there may not be anything worthwhile in the foods to begin with.

Nature provides fruits, vegetables, grains, and lean meat

for our nourishment. The further you get away from a natural-growing product with either leaves or hooves, the quicker you're ingesting something that offers no building blocks for your aging body. We are not getting any younger, and we need all the help we can receive from natural food to maintain health as long as possible. We need quantities of living foods—the fruits, vegetables, beans, and whole grains.

How many living foods have you eaten today? Living foods such as fruits, vegetables, grains, and nuts contain seeds that if planted can replicate another identical life form. Ingesting living foods breathes life into your body. Eating overly processed, dead foods provides no health benefits. Your body responds by dying one cell at a time, and disease begins from lack of "life." This is where the entire study of oxidants and antioxidants began. If you planted a prepackaged, well-preserved cookie into the soil, it would probably still be there five years from now. It has enough preservatives to keep it from rotting for years, but it certainly doesn't have any living nutrients to create another cookie. Even the insects will avoid it because they won't recognize it as food. Beware of what you are eating.

Supplements

Most of us take extra vitamins and minerals in pill form. Our soils are depleted in minerals, causing our foods to no longer offer the nutrition necessary to sustain complete health. Supplements help make up for the lack in our foods. If you rely only on supplements for nutrition, you're missing out on all the other good things you get from food. For example, foods high in vitamin C, such as green bell peppers and Brussel sprouts, are also rich in phytochemicals, which help fight cancer. Those same foods contain fiber, folate, and potassium. **The synergistic effect of nutrients and nonnutrient chemicals found together in living food helps fight diseases that try to invade our bodies.**

Bangles and Counting Servings

Our U.S. Government recommends that we eat at least 5 to 9 servings of vegetables and fruits daily. To help you remember how many servings you've eaten, wear bangles on your watch wrist each day, and as you eat one serving of a fruit or vegetable, move a bangle to the opposite wrist. It's a good reminder to use while you are developing better eating habits. You will find that your overall health will also improve.

Soluble and Insoluble Fiber

Both soluble and insoluble fiber help in preventing rectal cancer. Insoluble fiber found in whole grains speeds toxic elements through your intestines, whereas soluble fiber in fruits and vegetables removes tumor-promoting chemicals and creates compounds that can stop cancer cell growth.

White Bread Fattens Your Waistline

Of all the foods that digest quickly and zoom straight into your bloodstream as pure sugar, white bread has one of the highest ratings. Moreover, the sugar that isn't burned as energy gets stored as fat. Folks who eat four to five daily servings will see their waistlines widen quickly, and an inflated waist is a known heart-disease risk factor. Warning: switching to artificially colored "wheat" bread is just as bad for you. Whole-grain breads are heavy and can usually be found only in health-food stores. If the bread claims 100 percent whole wheat, that merely means it doesn't have rye, millet, corn or other grains added. Make sure it says 100 percent whole grain. In this case, the entire kernel of seed is used instead of filtering out all the rough and grainy parts.

Gout is Returning

Low-carb, high-protein diets promote a surge in cases of gout. That's because many foods eaten on these diets, especially red meats, contain purines—types of proteins that metabolize into uric acid. When the body produces too much uric acid or when the kidneys don't excrete enough of this waste product, the acid crystallizes in joints (most commonly the big toe) and causes pain and inflammation.

Gout is an inflammatory condition, so eating red, blue, or purple fruits every day —especially cherries, berries, or dark grapes—will cut the risk and the extent of the problem. Rich in antioxidants (cancer fighters), these fruits help reduce inflammation. Other methods are increasing your calcium intake, taking fish-oil supplements, adding omega-3s (oils that are essential for health), going light on high-purine animal foods such as meats, and watching what you drink. You need water, which helps dilute uric acid so it doesn't crystallize and cause pain.

Eat Yourself Young

Good eating habits will improve your health and slow down your aging process. Every day, the proven factor for longevity is in a healthy diet.

The Himalayan Hunza, the Vilcabamba of Ecuador, the Yucatan Mayan Indians, and people from remote regions of Bulgaria all have numerous members who live beyond one hundred years old. Not only do natives of these cultures live longer, most of them are free from many of the ailments that plague modernized societies—cancer, ulcers, indigestion, tooth decay, and senility.

Their high-fiber, low-fat diets consist of fresh fruits and vegetables, grains, and a good amount of proteins, such as beans, nuts, fish and extremely low-fat meats from free-roaming animals.

Trans Fats

Trans fats are bad for your heart. Called "partially hydrogenated" oils on food labels, trans fats raise the risk of a heart attack by clogging the arteries. **There are no safe levels of trans fats,** but the good news is that these unhealthy fats slowly disappear from your body over time once you stop eating them. Some of your favorite trans-fat foods are cake mixes, cereal and energy bars, chips and crackers, dried soups, frozen entrees, fast food, margarine, nondairy creamers and whipped toppings, packaged cookies, candy, donuts, pies, and cakes.

Your Vision

Fresh raw fruit can help prevent age-related macular degeneration. This condition appears in older people who do not eat fruits. Any kind of fresh raw fruit seems to help.

Need Fiber?

Fiber helps stabilize blood sugar and reduce cravings. A diet high in fiber reduces hunger. Fiber comes from eating real foods: fruits, vegetables, and whole-grain products. Fiber slows the digestion of carbohydrates, which prevents sudden changes in blood sugar levels that can cause hunger to return quickly. Fiber speeds the passage of food through the digestive tract, allowing less time for calories to be absorbed. As stored fat is burned, it often releases trapped toxins into our systems. These toxins can overload the liver, which plays a crucial role in breaking down fat, causing weight loss to stall. But if you're getting plenty of fiber, it will bind to many of the toxins and carry them out of the body, allowing the liver to function normally and more fat to melt away. Most Americans don't get even a small percentage of the daily fiber needed. This can be demonstrated in the waiting rooms of hospitals where more Americans have chronic cases of constipation every year. Colon cleansers are sadly lacking but desperately needed to clear the gunk out of our systems. If we returned to a high-fiber diet and stopped eating processed carbohydrates, disease would decrease at a phenomenal rate.

Body Waste

If you are not eliminating solid wastes from your bowels every day, you are not eating enough healthful, nutritious, fibrous foods or drinking enough water to flush your system. Frequent soft stool waste is essential to health; otherwise disease begins in the colon, where waste matter rots but is not being removed. Learn to listen to your body. Compacted and hurtful waste matter from your bowels is a warning that you need to heed. You may not be consuming enough fiber, or roughage, in your diet. Frequent use of laxatives can do more harm over time, as they flush away necessary minerals and irritate the linings of your intestines. Whole grains, green and yellow vegetables, white vegetables such as cauliflower, and raw fruits all contribute to the roughage needed to push mass through your colon in a reasonable amount of time.

If you only eliminate waste two or three times per week, you are setting yourself up for serious colon or intestinal diseases, as well as diverticulitis.

Constipation isn't exactly a pleasant topic of conversation, but it affects most people of all ages at some point in their lives. It seems to be a reflection of our modern, sedentary lifestyle. Various types of frequent constipation can lead to a more persistent condition if you don't catch these problems early. The accumulation of toxins in the large intestine can create an unhealthy environment conducive to headaches, bad breath, stomach aches, bloating, hemorrhoids, and other health problems. For more on this subject, please read Chapter 6: Death & Life Are in Your Colon.

Lack of abdominal muscle tone may be a cause of constipation for some. For example, people who sit at a desk all day, then sit for a long commute, go home, and sit in front of the TV all evening shouldn't be surprised if their abdominal muscles get lazy and their intestines need outside help to move things along. Walking helps. Vigorous walking purifies the blood by pumping more oxygen into the lungs and increasing blood circulation. It also improves digestion and stimulates intestinal muscular contractions that push waste along.

Fiber Helps Push Cholesterol Out

A diet high in fiber, such as that found in oats, beans, peas, barley, and raw pears, turns into a cholesterol magnet in your intestines, binding it up and escorting it out for elimination.

Whole-Grain Carbs Help You Stay Slim

High-fiber carbs such as heavy, whole-grain breads and whole-grain hot cereals burn more calories during digestion, help you feel full longer, and trigger less fat-storing insulin than refined carbs. The recommended amount of fiber per day is twenty-five to thirty-five grams. Most Americans don't come close to that figure, so you may need to plan some extra fiber into your menu until it becomes a habit.

Whole grains provide a fibrous seed coat and germ, where fiber and nutrients that prevent disease are found. **Refined grains in lightweight white and wheat breads offer only calories; the roughage and the most nutritious part of the grain (the seed germ) has been removed.**

If you search the cereal aisles of your local supermarket, you will find that hot cereals are much less expensive per serving and come in many varieties that can be sweetened with just a teaspoon of molasses or honey. Avoid the presweetened flavors. Homemade trail mix can be made using puffed wheat and corn or rice, and adding your favorite dried fruit and nut mix. Take it along with you on hikes, travels, or any adventure. These foods are high energy and loaded with vitamins and minerals.

Slow Carbs Slash Risk of Colon and Breast Cancers

Highly refined foods such as sugar and white flour are known as "fast" carbohydrates because they are digested too quickly.

Eating them makes your insulin levels spike, which can cause a metabolic disorder called insulin resistance. This condition is linked to heart disease and breast cancer.

Vegetarians: Low Protein and Zinc Levels Harm You

Protein stabilizes blood sugars, which reduces cravings and reduces the level of fat storage hormones. **The recommended dietary allowance of protein per day is from 0.4 to 0.5 grams per pound of weight.** In other words, if you weigh approximately two hundred pounds, you will need eighty to one hundred grams of protein per day to keep your cells functioning properly.

Some of us need more protein to feel full and satisfied. I'm one of those that need higher levels of protein each day (in the form of nuts, lean meats, and unsweetened yogurt) to feel satisfied and keep hunger away for hours.

Vegetarians, please take note: if you are not eating enough protein in beans or dairy products, you are probably protein-deficient. Your hair begins to fall out at a more rapid rate. Your nails break and split easily. Children who are forced to be non-dairy vegetarians are especially vulnerable to calcium- and protein-deficient diseases because they are growing so rapidly. Few vegetarian parents are properly educated to feed their children enough protein- and calcium-rich foods to keep them healthy. Children cannot maintain health on fruits, vegetables, bread, grains, and water. They need lots of protein from the bean groups if they are not eating meat, and children need quantities of calcium and protein to grow properly and develop healthy cells. I don't know very many children who eat three cups of cottage cheese or lentils daily.

Note the following list of protein sources with their grams of protein, and realize that you may need to eat the equivalent of **three to nine cups** of at least one of those sources daily to get enough protein in your diet, **depending on your weight** and what else you are eating. Since most food consumed has less protein than those listed below, you may well be a vegetarian who is protein-deficient.

Low-fat cottage cheese or ricotta cheese, 1 cup @ 28–29 grams

Soybeans, 1 cup @ 26 grams

Kidney, lima, black, navy beans, chickpeas, or split peas, 1 cup = 15–16 grams

Lentils, 1 cup @ 18 grams

Soy milk or soy yogurt, 1 cup @ 10–11 grams

1 veggie burger or veggie hot dog, 10 grams

Zinc deficiency is also one of the most common nutritional shortfalls among vegetarians. And that's unfortunate, because zinc deficiency can increase your risk of infection. Zinc is very important for the development of white blood cells, whose purpose is to recognize and destroy invading bacteria and viruses.

Vegetarians can also become deficient in vitamin B12, which treats fatigue, anxiety, memory loss, neuritis, hepatitis, and eye disorders, and is necessary for red blood cell formation. Sources are soybeans, eggs, pumpkin and squash seeds, wheat germ, yogurt, meat, and fish. How much of those meatless sources have you eaten daily?

Protein Holds Us Together

Protein is the stuff that holds us together. Structurally, proteins form your muscles, your skin tissues, and your ligaments. Internally, proteins make up your hormones, antibodies, blood, and enzymes. Every tissue that breaks down and needs repair needs protein, and since the body is constantly in need of repair and raw materials for growth, protein is essential to good health. Within one year, 98 percent of all the atoms in your body are replaced.

Proteins are constructed of amino acids, essential for nearly every body function. To work properly, proteins must be "complete," containing all eight essential amino acids. **Most complete proteins come from animals—meat, fish, eggs, and dairy products**. However, to make complete proteins from plant materials, you need to eat them in combination. Beans and rice or beans and corn dishes are found in virtually every culture.

I was a vegetarian for seven years and did not eat one forkful of meat or fish, but I had to eat more often because of hunger. Large amounts of beans or cottage cheese would only satisfy me for so long. It is possible to get enough protein from beans, cottage cheese, and legumes if you plan your meals properly and have no aversion to dairy products, but few people bother to research that carefully, and fewer adhere to a **high-protein vegetarian** lifestyle. It can be done, but please take care. At one point during my vegetarianism, I noticed my hair falling out at an accelerated rate—my first clue that I was becoming protein-deficient. Somewhere along the way, I shifted back to being a meat eater when I found that it satisfied my appetite more fully.

Women seem to have more of a problem with sugar cravings because of our fluctuating hormone levels during the month. **Eating enough protein will help you fend off those fattening urges**.

Allergies in Processed Foods

Many people have found to their dismay that they are extremely allergic to food dyes, MSG, and numerous other additives. Eat foods the way nature made them, and you will have fewer allergies and health problems. Shop in the raw produce section of your supermarket.

Before 1940, foods were closer to the way nature intended. Large amounts of sugar were not added to soups or BBQ sauce, and there was no fast food. I didn't see a McDonald's until I was twelve years old and visiting a large city in the Midwest. Meals were sit-down-and-stay-awhile dining experiences that you enjoyed three times per day with your family. They included protein, vegetables, fruit, a glass of milk, and a slice of whole-grain bread with nature-colored butter. Farmer's produce with fresh milk and eggs was an essential part of the community.

On our long family cross-country vacations, our parents fixed meals on the road. We ate sandwiches and drank cartons of milk or orange juice and fried eggs on the old camper stove. It cut travel expenses significantly for our large family. For snacks between meals, our parents would provide bags of fruit from road stands. The big treat for us was an occasional bottle of soda pop or a small ice cream cone. The one-scoop ice cream cones in 1950 were miniscule compared to today's mega-size scoops. I've had scoops of ice cream in recent years that would probably equal one pint per scoop. Swirled soft ice cream in the 1960s only rose about two or three inches above a three-inch cone. Today's soft swirled ice creams rise at least six inches above a six-inch cone, and then we wonder how we could have gained weight from that "one serving" size. Moreover, few people stop with such a simple order as plain ice cream. Today you can order your ice cream smothered with chocolate cookie crumbs or candy bar pieces or multicolored sugared sprinkles after a dip in chocolate syrup or a ladle of hot fudge. The calorie equivalent of such a delicacy might exceed what a normal person would eat in six meals.

During hot summer days as a teenager, I often rode my bicycle four miles to a tiny rural town, collecting cans and bottles from the ditches along the way for money from the bottle deposits to buy an ice cream cone upon arrival. The only flavors offered then were chocolate, strawberry, or vanilla, and store-bought ice cream was a delicious treat. We only ate the home-made hand-cranked variety at our house. Please note that in order to treat myself to that store-bought ice cream cone, I had to bike a round-trip of eight miles. Scoop sizes were almost bite size by today's standards. In that process, I probably burned off the entire serving before reaching home.

Even at an early age, I gravitated toward sweets when they were available. My grandfather would deliver a bag of cubed caramel candies once a month, and I ate them almost nonstop until the bag was empty. If the cookie jar was hollow, I baked more cookies to fill it. We were expected and required to eat three square meals per day—all prepared entirely from scratch. Pancake and biscuit batters were mixed with whole-grain flours and fresh raw milk and eggs. Noodles were hand-made by rolling out a large round pad of dough and slicing it into noodle-sized strips. There were no prepackaged foods in our home. Our animals were butchered for meat, while fruits and vegetables were raised and preserved by the sweat of our brow.

Only the hard work of farming and caring for farm animals kept my weight somewhat in check. We were in excellent physical condition, and our parents did not differentiate between my brothers or sisters when it came to doing hard labor. We worked at shoveling feed, forking silage to our cattle, milking cows, hauling feed to the chickens, and tossing bales of hay to the livestock, in addition to seeding and weeding the garden, picking the apples and plums from the orchard, and freezing and canning the food for preservation. In the summertime, between our evening and morning chores or other essential farm activities, I rode my bicycle several miles per day for fun or walked around the farm section—(four miles) in just an hour. In nice weather, the outdoors beckoned and I couldn't stay inside. There were butterflies to chase, the old black dog to romp with, horses to ride, and the tire hanging from the old sycamore tree in the backyard to swing on.

One high school summer I worked at the local "bee house" in town, where we removed combs of honey from the heavy hive boxes brought into the plant and placed them into huge spinning tanks that separated the honey from the combs. That job required us to stand, bend, and lift eight hours per day. The liquid honey flowed into giant five-gallon cans for transport. Our large family would generally use an entire five-gallon can of honey every year. We used it as a sweetener for our cereal and poured spoonfuls of it on home-baked bread and pancakes. During that particular summer, I was also biking eight miles round-trip daily to my place of work. During this same summer, I had to keep up with the farm chores morning and night at home. This was also the summer that I crash-dieted by eating only six hundred calories per day and lost three pounds per week for four months and almost killed myself from malnutrition. What frustrated me the most was the fact I was doing all that and only lost three pounds per week (which is faster than the recommended healthy weight loss).

As you can ascertain, my early years did not revolve around sedentary activities such as sitting in front of a television or computer screen (Bill Gates hadn't invented the desktop computer yet). My parents didn't even bring a television into the house until I was in my later years of high school, toward the end of the 1960s.

Foods Other Than Sweets

While you are eating the various food groups each day, seriously consider whether fruits or breads cause you to overeat. Diabetics especially have to consider the glycemic levels in foods. For high and low glycemic foods, check out the website: diabetes.ca/Section_About/glycemic.asp. Starchy foods such as potatoes, peas, or corn have a higher glycemic level. Eating too many foods with higher glycemic numbers will greatly reduce your ability to lose weight and will interfere with your insulin levels. If you eat four bread rolls with your dinner each day, you probably are addicted to something in those ingredients. Instead, get your grains from hot cooked cereals or switch to a heavier and healthier variety of whole-grain bread that doesn't tempt you to overeat but fills you with fiber. When it takes more time to chew, it will slow down your "gulping mode" and you will feel full after one slice. If you only splurge on white rolls several times a year at major holiday dinners, then rolls probably aren't a problem for you.

Fruit

If fruit causes you to overeat, increase your proteins and vegetables and choose lower glycemic-index fruits that don't trigger your overeating responses. Blueberries and other berries have tremendous amounts of antioxidants (the thing that keeps cells from turning into cancer cells). If cherries or grapes cause your blood sugar levels to skyrocket or cause you to overeat, then switch to a type of fruit that works for you. Abandon fruit drinks containing sugar, fructose, or corn syrup. Please don't feed them to your children. If something is not healthy for you, it definitely is not healthy for a growing child. The real fruit with all its fiber will keep you feeling satisfied and feed your body nutritiously. Look for juice that is 100 percent juice, with no additives, sugars, or dyes, and don't use over one or two servings of fruit juice per day. You only need *a half cup of juice to equal one fruit serving.* Use your twenty-ounce glassware for water or unsweetened tea. Beware of canned fruits that have unhealthy amounts of added sugars. Eating these will also increase your appetite and raise your insulin levels. It's better to avoid those and stick with raw, untainted fruit that grows naturally as God intended. One whole orange will satisfy your appetite longer with its fiber, then a half cup of orange juice. Too much juice can cause gas and tummy aches, especially in children. You may want to dilute their juice with water. You may find that you can't drink juice with a meal or you'll experience heartburn.

The key to better health is returning to natural, unprocessed foods.

Let Me Regress Again

You have probably tried dozens of diets and failed miserably, or you wouldn't be reading this book. Those of us who are over the half-centurion mark did not drink sodas on a daily basis in childhood. We drank fluids that nourished our cells: milk or raw orange juice or just plain water and lots of it. We sat down to home-cooked meals together, and we always ate a large breakfast. We ate huge quantities of home-baked, whole-grain bread with volumes of honey, jam, and butter between meals because we had huge appetites and were very active farm people. We worked hard. We played hard, and we ate in proportion to our activity level.

Dessert was offered after all the meat, vegetables, and fruits were consumed off the table. Dessert was more like an afterthought and sometimes not served until one or two hours after dinner or forgotten altogether. This gave ample time for the evening meal to settle. We were able to burn off all those calories.

It's been noted that the Amish people actually consume about the same amount of calories as the average American, but their activity level is so much higher than average that the high level of obesity is not found amongst them as it is in the rest of the populace. The Amish generally eat fewer processed foods and therefore are eating more fibrous, natural foods that don't become fodder for their fat-storing cells.

Today, typical inactive Americans choose to make a meal around a supersized milk shake or soda drink that could drown a small dog and which already contains a day's worth of calories. A typical American will eat four huge slices of pizza at a single meal, down a twenty-ounce Coke, and wonder why he is hungry again long before his next meal. Then he spends ten to twelve hours per day sitting at a desk job, sitting at lunch with co-workers, and sitting while commuting back and forth to work. Are we seeing a problem here?

There are now supersized burgers with buns that contain anywhere from 1,200 to 1,400 calories. Today's muffins are the size of cakes and should be divided up to feed a starving family, not served as a snack for one individual. Over half a century ago, home-baked muffins and cornbread were not sweet. You added a spoonful of honey or jelly when the muffins came fresh from the oven if you desired a sweeter taste. Today, there is more sugar in a monster muffin than there used to be in an average-sized, home-baked cupcake, which was less than half the size of today's muffin. There are enough calories in a supersized drink and a massive burger to fill the entire quota of daily calories for a six-foot, four-inch 250-pound muscle-bound man. But where is the nutrition? Except for the protein in the burger, the rest is mostly empty calories. There is no fruit, and the only vegetable is a slice of wilted lettuce that has almost zero nutrition, or a thin slice of tomato that was picked green over a month ago and its vitamins have long since evaporated. The bun is made from overprocessed bleached flour that no self-respecting bug would touch.

Whole Grains

Whole grains have been removed from most varieties of bread today, so grain-depleted white breads or "artificially colored wheat" breads made from enriched bleached flours give your body no nutrition. These are empty, wasted calories. Your cells are screaming for wholesome foods, because they are getting almost zero nutrition and no building blocks to repair cell damage. Your white blood cells aren't finding enough nutrients to divide and multiply to fight the daily invasion of germs in your body, so your immune system falters. So guess what? You eat more. And you are constantly coming down with colds and flu-like symptoms. Most Americans continue to make wrong feeding choices. They stuff themselves full of highly processed, plastic foods that have little or no nutritional value and wonder why they are constantly hungry, depressed, anxious, sick with colds or sore throats, or lack energy. We sit on our couches by the hour, pressing the remote buttons, too lethargic to move more than our index finger. We have time for mindless programs but no time to maintain our health. Chapter 4 discusses the importance of nutrition. You may find what your body is missing.

The breads that my mother baked could have been used for weapons of war. They were heavy enough to do serious bodily damage if thrown at your opposition. The average loaf of bread sold in the supermarket today could bounce off your skull without notice.

We had the advantage of raising our own grains when I was growing up. Our wheat grinder was hooked to a motor, so we had freshly ground wheat, corn, and rye flours with all the enzymes and parts intact to make our bread. You could even say we were a bit fanatical about eating healthier foods, but I am so thankful that my parents gave us that very healthy start in life.

My mother always raised huge amounts of fresh garden vegetables every summer and canned and froze packages by the thousands to feed our large family all winter long. We churned butter from the heavy cream that rose to the top of the milk from our own dairy cattle, and we drank unlimited amounts of raw, nonfat milk (with the cream removed).

Though we cannot go back to the past (I now live in the suburbs, as do most of you), I have found heavier and grainier types of breads in health-food shops nearby. The taste will beat anything you'd find at your supermarket, and one slice toasted and spread with cream cheese or old-fashioned peanut butter (free from hydrogenated oil, which clogs your arteries) will fill you up and provide you with one or two servings of a whole-grain product. After you've eaten a slice, you will feel like you've eaten something substantial and will be quite satisfied. It also helps in moving body wastes out to avoid constipation.

Today's Chickens

Growing up on a farm I have an advantage to compare today's commercially sold foods to what is grown naturally.

Free-range chickens (chickens that are free to roam around a grass-filled yard, instead of being raised in small cages) are not marbled with fat. I'm rather shocked when I eat the usual store-bought chicken or KFC and find globs of yellow, greasy fat hanging from the meat. No wonder our cholesterol levels have increased. One solution is to buy your meats from stores that specialize in free-range animals, or broil your meat so the fat runs off harmlessly into the pan instead of into your body.

Head Off a Stroke

Take off pounds if you're overweight. Eat a diet low in saturated fat and cholesterol.

Cut out alcohol. Even small amounts can lead to large changes in triglyceride levels. Be physically active for at least thirty minutes, five days a week. Use canola oil, olive oil, or sugar-free peanut butter with no trans fats. Cut back on simple carbohydrate intake (desserts made with processed sugars and flours). Eat more fatty fish, such as salmon, tuna, mackerel, and sardines, because they're high in beneficial omega-3 fatty acids, but in moderation because of possible mercury contamination.

Choose to Lose

We can't return to the past, but we can make wiser choices today. Healthy, nutritional, and vibrant living foods are available, if you make the effort to find them. Many health food stores include whole-grain choices of cereals, breads,organic fruits and vegetables. Community Supported Agriculture groups (CSAs) are springing up across America. Remove processed sugars while learning to enjoy the taste of real food. Your increasing health will be your reward.

Chapter 4

Vitamins, Minerals, and Other Essentials

"Change your thinking to change your life."

MY FIRST SERIOUS DIET occurred at age fourteen when my weight rose to 156 pounds. I crash-dieted for fourteen weeks on six hundred calories per day to lose about three pounds a week to reach 112 pounds. I was so nutritionally deprived afterward that the only way I could get any energy was to eat as much as possible. I ate to gain back my strength and feel better physically. Though I felt just fine while losing the weight, the aftereffects slowed me for years. Just climbing stairs or trying to be active made me exhausted, and I was as weak as a sick cat without being sick. That extreme starvation diet left me very tired and deprived of essential nutrients. It took several years to replace the essential missing nutrients before my health rebounded. At that time, not as much was known about nutrition. As a teenager, reading about vitamins and minerals never crossed my mind. It did take about two years to regain the full forty-four pounds because of the active lifestyle I was living.

We Need Nutrition Knowledge

When I was in my thirties, both of my forearms began hurting. It came on very gradually, until it was painful to bend my wrists and elbows. Somewhere I had read the importance of vitamin C in reducing bone aches. At that time in my life, I had been leaving out citrus fruit and it showed. Remember the sailors and how they developed scurvy because they were on board ship for so many months without any vitamin C? Their solution was to transport limes and ingest the lime juice during long voyages, hence solving their scurvy problem. Once I returned to the habit of eating either one citrus fruit (oranges or grapefruit) or drinking one glass of 100 percent orange juice every day, those aches in my arms disappeared within three days.

About that same time in my life, I became quite weepy when there was nothing different going on. There was no trauma happening to me. My life was continuing along at a fairly stable pace. There was no emotional reason to have these weepy times. After studying certain nutritional deficiencies and their effects, it dawned on me that my hormones were probably changing with my advancing age. Again, nutrition solved the problem: I increased my vitamin B. As long as I took a daily supply of soluble (easily absorbed) vitamin B and sprinkled wheat germ on my cereal each morning, the weeping episodes disappeared. If I forgot to take supplements for several days, the weeping returned.

Below are some important facts about essential nutrients.

Calcium

Your life can be extended by increasing your calcium intake and absorption. Without enough calcium, the functioning of every cell in your body breaks down. Oranges and dairy products such as milk, cheese, cottage cheese, or yogurt have adequate amounts of calcium to prevent calcium deficiencies but only if consumed in large amounts.

Calcium is required all our lives for bones, teeth, muscle, nerve function, and blood clotting. Muscle pains, cramps, twitches, and even convulsions may suggest calcium deficiency.

Most of us have calcium deficiencies, and if we would all get maximum amounts of absorption of calcium into our bodies, many of our diseases would vaporize and our quality of life would improve. Take the recommended dosage of vitamin D and calcium, which work in conjunction with each other, to insure proper absorption into your body where it can be utilized.

When the body does not get enough calcium, it will withdraw what little calcium it has from the bones to make sure that there is a steady supply in the bloodstream. **As the body does its best to compensate for the deficiency, it builds bony deposits and spurs to reduce movement and limit activity.**

Premenopausal symptoms such as cramps and hot flashes have long been associated with calcium deficiencies.

Menopause is a natural part of life, not something to dread. If your body is doing strange things at this important time in your life, listen to it. Perhaps it is out of sync because you have neglected yourself for years in lack of exercise, lack of calcium, or poor eating habits. Educate yourself and make the necessary changes; your health is all that stands between you and your quality of life. Many healthy women sail through menopause with no hot flashes, no cramps, and no discomfort of any kind. A healthy body is designed by our Creator to handle hormonal changes.

No other mineral is capable of performing as many biological functions as calcium. This amazing mineral provides the electrical energy for the heart to beat and for all muscle movement. It is the calcium ion that is responsible for feeding every cell. Another important biological job for calcium is DNA replication, which is crucial for maintaining youth and a healthy body. Thus, **low calcium means low body repair and premature aging**. Calcium is the big player in pH control. Calcium quickly destroys oxygen-robbing acid in the body fluids. With low calcium in your body, more cancer and other degenerative diseases strike.

The heart's ability to contract and beat rhymatically would not be possible without calcium.

Calcium and Vitamin D Fight Colon Cancer

Both calcium and vitamin D discourage growth of noncancerous tumors that are forerunners to colorectal cancer. Most American diets fall short on vitamin D. If milk is your only source, you need four eight-ounce glasses to get enough. Although yogurt and cheese are calcium-packed, they have zero vitamin D. Sunshine will give you vitamin D for free, or you can also take the recommended dosage daily in a multivitamin if you are simply unable to get outside on most sunny days.

Sunlight and Vitamin D

Without vitamin D, most of the ionized calcium would pass through the body. Vitamin D comes from sunlight. It should also be noted that light entering the eyes influences many of your glands, which control the entire endocrine system, including the calcium-regulating glands.

Unfortunately, most folks today spend the majority of their lives under artificial lighting that does not have the full spectrum lighting that our bodies need. When "full-spectrum" lighting is used, human calcium absorption increases, plants flourish, and cows produce more milk. Full-spectrum lighting is used to treat psoriasis, neonatal jaundice, and herpes simplex infections. Tinted glass can eliminate a large percentage of the sun's light spectrum and therefore affects you both physically and psychologically. Grandma knew that kids were healthier if they got fresh air, sunshine, and good food.

Sun on the skin regulates mineral disposition in the body and produces vitamin D, which allows the intestine to absorb large amounts of nutrients and raises the pH of body fluids. This helps in preventing and curing disease. Lack of sunshine on the body is responsible for a host of diseases, especially cancer. There is twice as much breast cancer in the northern states as in the sunny southern states. Prostate cancer almost triples from the sunny Mexican border to the northern Canadian border.

Sunlight is good for your health. Unfortunately, artificial light sources have made a major change for the worse in human lifestyles. It is now possible to work and live without natural sunlight but at great risk to health. Your body needs unfiltered sunlight **to regulate your appetite, sleep, body temperature, sexual functions, water balance, and hormones**. All living things need to be exposed daily to sunlight. Try to get quality unfiltered sunlight on your skin each day, but never stay in the sun long enough to become sunburned. Too much of anything can be dangerous to your health.

Seasonal Affective Disorder (SAD)

SAD, a reaction to reduced sunlight during the shorter days of winter, creates the urge to snack on high-sugar, highly refined foods. You can beat your blues by soaking up natural light on daily walks or investing in a natural-spectrum lamp that emulates natural light to give you a feeling of well-being. I use a full-spectrum lamp for projects in my basement and forget all about being underground. One of my co-workers keeps a tiny full-spectrum light on her desk to help conquer her SAD since the tinted windows keep out the natural sunlight.

Living Under the Redwoods

For a dozen years I lived under the giant redwoods of coastal California near Santa Cruz. The sun barely penetrated through the forest to allow sunlight. The only hanging plants that flourished in that dark environment were shade-lovers such as ferns and ivy. On sunny days, I hiked a mile to our local state park where an entrance road ran through a large, open meadow, just to escape the dark, shady dampness of the trees and soak up sunlight. I craved sunlight in this environment and went out of my way to find it. On weekends, I drove to the open beach along the Pacific Ocean just to expose my face to the open sky and bright light. During one particularly long rainy season, I opened my car door to find mushrooms growing in the heavy carpet on the floorboard. I used to call living under the redwoods "dark, damp, and dripping." Several of our neighbors had full-spectrum lighting" installed in rooms where they gathered the most to keep their sanity intact in this almost cavelike existence.

One time my sister and husband visited and stayed in a cabin several miles down the road within the redwood forest. We planned to venture out early one morning, but they didn't arrive until two hours late—unusual as they were normally early risers. I didn't even have to ask what happened. It was so dark under those trees that they overslept.

Sunlight produces and regulates vitamin D and therefore is essential in the maintenance of strong, healthy bones. Lack of vitamin D brings about rickets, which still affects children in certain areas of the world where their bones fail to absorb calcium, phosphorous, and other minerals to make them hard and strong. As a result, the bones bend and deform. Rickets can be both prevented and cured by a few minutes per day in strong sunlight. Adults can suffer loss of bone mineral and weakening of their bones, a disorder called osteomalacia. Exposure to sunlight will reverse this problem. Unfortunately, senior citizens in nursing homes all too often don't get enough natural sunlight to keep their bones strong. All senior citizen buildings should have built-in solariums where residents can soak up natural sunlight in any weather or season.

Never let your skin burn. Be sensible about the amount

of time you spend in the sun. Vitamin D can actually retard the growth and spread of malignant melanoma cells. Vitamin D slows the growth and development of breast cancer, colon cancer, and prostate cancer.

Since the incidences of breast, colon, and prostate cancer are lowest in the sunny countries near the equator and increase as you move northward, it's obvious that exposure to sunlight must help diminish these diseases.

Another surprising result from lack of sunlight occurs in vague, chronic aches in various areas of your body. If you have chronic pain or fibromyalgia, ask your family doctor to test your blood level of vitamin D. Sometimes the simplest of solutions may be to get a few minutes of sunlight every day.

Multiple Sclerosis and Sunlight

Virtually no cases of multiple sclerosis are found near the equator, and the rate increases rapidly the further north you travel: more sunlight, less multiple sclerosis. However, never allow yourself to burn or you set yourself up for skin cancers. Skin cells are broken down by burning.

People who consume artificial sweeteners in everything from diet sodas to fruit-flavored yogurt and bubblegum can exhibit symptoms very similar to multiple sclerosis.

Omega-3s Found in Plants as Well as Fish

Omega-3 fats are essential for heart health. Omega-3s are found in flaxseed oil, canola oil, walnut oil, soybeans, walnuts, fish, and tofu. Nowadays, the concern over mercury-poisoned fish causes many people to seek alternative sources of omega-3s.

Nuts and Seeds Are Essential to Health

All nuts and seeds contain nutrients to begin new life. If planted, they will sprout into another seed-bearing plant containing the essentials to create life. Nuts and seeds feed your body life in ways that pump oxygen into your cells. Your cells cannot function properly without these important minerals and vitamins. Each nut or seed (almonds, cashews, Brazil nuts, pecans, peanuts, walnuts, pumpkin seeds, sunflower seeds, and so on) contains many if not most of the following: high fiber, potassium, phosphorus, calcium, magnesium, selenium, iron, zinc, manganese, copper, niacin, folate, and vitamins A, C, E, and K.

Almonds and sunflower seeds also contain large amounts of vitamin E.

Walnuts, pecans, pistachios, and hazelnuts are high in heart-helping omega-3 fatty acids, which help stabilize your heartbeat to prevent potentially fatal irregularities called arrhythmias.

If you don't particularly care for fish, nuts will also give you essential oils.

The healthy fat in nuts slows vision-robbing macular degeneration and lowers LDL cholesterol.

The fiber in nuts keeps people from gaining as much weight because it takes longer to digest and helps you feel fuller. The consumption of nuts has been proven to lower your body's production of triglycerides.

Unfortunately, people have been brainwashed into believing that nuts should be avoided because they are high in calories. Yes, nuts are high in calories and fats, but those calories, fats, enzymes, and nutrients are essential to your health, and a small handful of nuts have far fewer calories than a damaging slice of cake or pie that goes straight to your hips and deteriorates your health on the way. The healthy fats, fiber, and protein in nuts are so filling that you will actually eat less.

Healthy Heart Cuisine

Fruits are important health sources that have received a bad rap by dieters who count calories. We've been taught that eating fruit is bad for us because of higher calories.

May I ask, higher calories compared to what? Each fruit is loaded with sustaining nutrients for our bodies, as well as necessary fiber. Compare that to a slice of nonnutrient, nonfilling, nonfiber chocolate-iced cake or a bowlful of ice cream at four hundred to eight hundred calories. The average apple, banana, or orange contains only about 100 calories each and is loaded with fiber, minerals, and vitamins essential to your health. Are you going to replace that with one scoop of ice cream, one slice of white bread, or an entire package of chocolate chip cookies? Who are you fooling? Junk foods are loaded with sugar and no nutrients, so you become hungry in ten minutes and want more of the same without quenching your hunger or supplying what your body needs. **When your body is starving for nutrients, it will keep your hunger switch on high.**

Fruit fiber is very filling and has higher water content and fewer calories than other fattening carbohydrates, so you're more likely to feel full after eating it. Because it is a complex carbohydrate instead of a simple sugar, it does not go straight to your hips.

Fruits have most of the following: potassium, calcium, phosphorus, magnesium, selenium, iron, manganese, copper, zinc, and vitamins A, B (avocados), C, and E. Even bananas have niacin. Fruits are loaded with nutrients that prevent cancers and squelch free radicals. Just for example, one cup of blackberries contains protein, fiber, potassium, calcium, phosphorus, magnesium, manganese, iron, selenium, zinc, folate, and vitamins A, C, and E and traces of copper.

Those who eat many servings of fruits and vegetables per day have less risk of most cancers and tumors. Citrus fruits cut your risk of mouth, throat, and stomach cancers.

Papayas, Mangos, and Bananas are Immune System Boosters

Tropical fruits have many antiaging benefits. Bananas are full of magnesium, which protects circulatory function while helping prevent hypoglycemia and blood-sugar swings.

Papayas are loaded with enzymes that help the body fight off infections while strengthening the immune system and reducing the effects of allergies.

Mangos have phytochemicals that act as antioxidants and immune system boosters.

Bananas and Artichoke Leaves

The potassium levels so richly contained in bananas and artichoke leaves coats and soothes the stomach lining and lowers acid overproduction, reducing painful gas and heartburn.

Blueberries and the Brain

Chemicals in blueberries block cholesterol from penetrating into the brain blood vessels, which requires proper blood flow for mental energy and health.

Cherries Are a Natural Painkiller

To alleviate pain from arthritis, eat six to eight cherries a day. Cherries are good sources of minerals like magnesium (a natural painkiller) and potassium (a natural diuretic), reducing inflammation by ridding tissue of excess fluid.

Figs Shrink Tumors

Figs and fig extracts contain the compounds that can successfully shrink tumors in humans. Figs have long been used as a poultice to draw out the poison in boils.

Wrinkle Protection

Loading up on red, yellow, and orange fruits and vegetables packs your skin with carotenoids, helping protect you from sunburn, wrinkles, and skin cancer.

Carotenoids work like a layer of sunscreen. The more you consume, the greater the protection. Carotenoid-rich foods are cantaloupe, mango, papaya, and tomatoes. Still important, though: don't stay in the sun long enough to burn.

Strawberries and Grapes for Treating Cancer

Strawberries and grapes are especially good sources found effective in preventing and treating cancer of the esophagus.

Avocado Lovers

Avocados are a great source of monounsaturated fat (known to keep cholesterol levels down). They are loaded with vitamin E, making them the highest fruit source of this powerful antioxidant. Avocados also help reduce prostate cancer cell growth and protect against cataracts and macular degeneration. People who are concerned about their high calorie content need to just enjoy the occasional benefits of this very special fruit. Eating any healthy food in moderation is of greater benefit than avoiding it altogether. Avocados certainly have fewer calories than dessert, which causes damage to your body.

Vegetables

Most vegetables are loaded with potassium, phosphorus, magnesium, calcium, selenium, iron, manganese, copper, and zinc, as well as vitamin A and C, niacin, and folate.

Breast Cancer Flees From Broccoli

Here is one more healthy reason to eat your broccoli, cabbage, Brussels sprouts, and cauliflower: these vegetables contain nutrients that **prevent changes that can lead to cancer in human breast cells** and **halt the growth of malignant breast cells.**

Menstrual Migraines and Magnesium

Magnesium deficiency has been linked with migraines. Your best sources are nuts and leafy greens.

Tomatoes Stop Many Cancers

The antioxidants abundant in tomatoes have been shown to cut the risk of prostate, colorectal, lung, breast, and cervical cancers. However, if you have arthritis inflammation, avoid this member of the nightshade family, as well as bell peppers, potatoes, and eggplants; your joints will ache worse from their toxins.

Oatmeal

Oatmeal really is good for you. Not only have oats been shown to be a cholesterol-lowering food, but the fiber and complex carbohydrates in this grain can keep you going. One of the main causes of a midmorning slump is that your body just runs out of fuel a few hours after breakfast. When your morning begins with high-calorie junk food, you can really feel your energy lag after the sugar has metabolized. But oats are different because of high fiber. The complex carbohydrates in oatmeal fill you up and metabolize slowly, releasing controlled energy throughout the morning. So, by the time you get to lunch, you'll still be going strong.

Beans are Anticancer Agents

A staple for many indigenous peoples around the world, beans are not only good for your heart, they help provide much-needed fiber, protein, and complex carbohydrates for general nutrition and are used as anticancer agents.

Beans can stimulate colon bacteria to lower cholesterol, reduce blood pressure, and lessen the risk of colon cancer.

Garlic and Onions

Garlic can add years to your life because it fights infection, reduces the risk of cancer, thins the blood, stimulates the immune system, reduces rates of blood clotting, and even lowers blood pressure. Cancer has also been shown to back up in the presence of garlic. My father is living proof that garlic and onions can help you lead a long life. He smoked for almost forty years and drank heavily the last forty years of his life, and he still had a sharper mind and better health when he died at ninety than most folks his age. He ate garlic and onions almost daily.

Onions can lower cholesterol, thin the blood, and reduce blood pressure.

Mushrooms

Mushrooms increase the production and activity of white blood cells, making them more aggressive—a good thing when you have an infection.

Spinach Benefits

Spinach can lower blood cholesterol.

Carrots Reduce Lung Cancer Risk

Carrots not only help reduce the lung cancer risk in smokers, but they reduce the risk of cancer in ex-smokers and people exposed to cigarette smoke as well. Beta-carotene seems to be the key. This nutrient seems to stop the formation of cancer in its later stages.

Asparagus for Energy

This vegetable is loaded with nutrients essential for energy, including potassium, phosphorous, and calcium.

Olive Oil and Heart Health

The health of the people in Mediterranean countries is a great testament to the heart-smart benefits of olive oil. People have been using olive oil for so long, no one knows exactly where or when they first began. People in Crete eat more olive oil than any other population in the world. They also have one of the world's lowest incidences of heart disease and cancer.

Olive oil's main benefit is that it lowers "bad" LDL cholesterol, while raising the blood levels of "good" HDL cholesterol. It also thins the blood, reducing the risk of clots and strokes.

Celery for Arthritis

Celery is a diuretic, and the loss of excess fluid can reduce the inflammation associated with arthritis without using drugs that may have harmful side effects.

Eggs Improve Cholesterol Levels

Eating whole eggs may significantly improve your cholesterol levels—even if your levels usually rise when eating other cholesterol-rich foods! It's difficult to get choline without eating eggs and butter. Choline is vital to human health in that it reduces cholesterol, promotes learning and memory, and reduces symptoms of menopause.

Fatty Acids

Not all fats are bad. Your body cannot be healthy without omega-3 fats.

Your body uses essential fatty acids for a number of important functions. Fatty acids control your body temperature; regulate inflammation, swelling, and pain; and are involved in blood clotting, allergic reactions, and hormone production. In the days before refined vegetable oils, people got their essential fatty acids from whole grains, nuts, vegetables, and egg yolks. Today the average American consumes large amounts of refined corn, soy, safflower, and canola oils, which are extra high in omega-6 fatty acids. People eat very little omega-3 fatty acids derived from fish, egg yolks, nuts, nut oils, and whole grains. This, along with the widespread use of trans fats, results in heart disease, cancer, inflammatory ailments, autoimmune illnesses, and other chronic, degenerative conditions.

Breakfast Makes Champions

Make breakfast or lunch your largest meal. You burn calories faster and more completely one hour after you wake up than at any other time of the day. The single best dieting strategy is to eat a big meal before 9:00 AM every day, even if you aren't accustomed to eating a sizable breakfast. Getting in the habit of eating a light dinner and a large breakfast will help you maintain your blood sugar levels all day, while not storing mass amounts of fat at night.

Wine and Grape Juice

The health benefits of red wine have been toted for years as protecting against certain cancers and heart disease, lowering cholesterol levels, and reducing blood pressure. Excessive or binge drinking, however, doesn't produce the same benefits. In other words, when it comes to drinking alcoholic beverages, **more is not better**. The compounds responsible for healing are the antioxidants.

One thing that wine lovers are not told is that 100 percent purple grape juice has the same health benefits as its fermented cousin, without the destructive path that often leads to alcoholism.

Common Vitamins, Treatments, and Sources

Vitamin A

Vitamin A reduces risk of measles, boosts the immune system, helps wounds heal, promotes good eyesight, and helps skin resist infection. Sources are apricots, asparagus, beans, carrots, citrus fruits, squash, yogurt, milk, carrots, sweet potatoes, and liver.

Vitamin B1 (Thiamin)

Thiamin treats stress, depression, hangovers, motion sickness, shingles, and neuralgia and is essential for carb metabolization. Sources are grains, beans, corn, figs, green peas, egg yolks, and liver.

Vitamin B2 (Riboflavin)

Riboflavin is used to treat depression, anxiety, stress disorders, carpal tunnel, and eye problems and is essential for protein metabolism and skin and eye protection. Sources are almonds, broccoli, green leafy vegetables, wheat germ, yogurt, milk, mushrooms, meat, and poultry.

Vitamin B3 (Niacin)

Niacin is used to treat high cholesterol, alcoholism, migraines, anxiety, arthritis, and schizophrenia. Sources are nuts, fish, meat, and poultry.

Vitamin B5 (Pantothenic Acid)

This acid treats allergies, weak adrenal glands, ulcers, anxiety, depression, hypoglycemia, and eczema, postpones graying of hair, assists in the synthesis of important steroids and cholesterols, and helps metabolize nutrients. Sources are beans, molasses, nuts, yeast, liver, eggs, certain vegetables, whole grains, and wheat germ.

Vitamin B6

Vitamin B6 treats PMS, acne, depression, diabetes, carpal tunnel syndrome, and anemia and is important in regulating the nervous system. You can find this vitamin in whole grains, nuts, meat, bananas, and wheat germ.

Vitamin B12

Vitamin B12 treats fatigue, anxiety, memory loss, neuritis, hepatitis, eye disorders, and is necessary for red blood cell formation. Sources are soybeans, eggs, meat, and fish.

Vitamin B15

Vitamin B15 helps eliminate body toxins, uses antioxidant action to protect against cancer, and lowers cholesterol. Sources are bran, brown rice, pumpkin seeds, sesame seeds, and whole grains.

Vitamin C

This multipurpose vitamin treats cancer, immune problems, cardiovascular disease, diabetes, gallstones, eye problems, allergies, and asthma.

Lack of Vitamin C in your food increases your risk of heart attacks and atherosclerosis. An abundance of Vitamin C reduces your chances of getting cancers of the stomach, esophagus, colon, bladder, cervix, uterus, and breast. Enjoy your citrus fruits.

A century ago, fewer than half of all Americans saw the other side of sixty-five. After sixty-five, women faced double the risk of stroke. People with the highest vitamin C intake are considerably less likely to have a stroke than are those with the lowest intake. Even smokers are able to cut their stroke rate by consuming large amounts of vitamin C. Boost your intake with red bell peppers, sliced kiwi, orange sections (not just the juice), Brussels sprouts, and strawberries. Vitamin C is found in all fruits and vegetables, with larger amounts in the citrus fruit family, bell peppers, and tomatoes.

Vitamin D

This treats menopausal symptoms, poor calcium absorption, and brittle bones. These chronic symptoms can be relieved with small amounts of sunlight every day. Sources are milk, cheese, egg yolk, cod liver oil, sunlight, and tuna.

Vitamin E

Vitamin E slows heart disease and wards off memory problems associated with aging. By preventing the formation of damaging free radicals in your body, vitamin E can help protect against brain cell damage, anemia, immune diseases, and DNA damage that leads to cancer or premature aging. Women going through menopause can especially benefit from vitamin E supplements because estrogen, often taken to lessen the symptoms of menopause, can cause vitamin E deficiencies.

Wheat germ is one of the best natural sources of this important vitamin. Available in the cereal aisle of most supermarkets, wheat germ can be sprinkled on food. I add wheat germ and flax powder to my hot cereal in the morning. Other natural sources of vitamin E are green vegetables, whole grains, wheat germ oil, almonds, sunflower seeds, eggs, and soybeans.

Vitamin K

Lack of this vitamin is most often associated with nosebleeds and morning sickness. Vitamin K helps clot blood, wards off osteoporosis, and reduces the risk of cancer. Sources are tomatoes, green leafy vegetables, cabbage, and broccoli.

Beta-carotene

Beta-carotene treats lung cancer and increases the ability of the immune system to fight disease. Sources are broccoli, Brussels sprouts, carrots, grapefruit, green leafy vegetables, mango, papaya, and squash.

Biotin

Biotin treats eczema, diabetes, and dialysis problems and helps hair growth. Sources are liver, egg yolk, milk, fruit, nuts, and yeast.

Choline

This ingredient reduces cholesterol, improves neurotransmitter activity, promotes memory and learning, reduces symptoms of menopause, and benefits your kidneys, liver, and heart. Sources are eggs, bran, green leafy vegetables, organ meats, and wheat germ.

Folic Acid

This acid treats canker sores, heart disease, psoriasis, and pernicious anemia; helps prevent birth defects; reduces cervical dysplasia in women who take oral contraceptives; improves mental function; and stimulates formation of red blood cells. Sources are green plants, fresh fruits, liver, yeast, egg yolks, carrots, and cantaloupe.

Common Minerals, Treatments, and Sources

Calcium

This all-important mineral works with phosphorus and vitamin D to form strong bones and teeth. Calcium eases insomnia and helps regulate the passage of nutrients through cell walls. Without calcium, your muscles won't contract correctly, your blood won't clot, and your nerves won't carry messages. Without enough calcium, your body automatically takes calcium from your bones—without adequate replacement; as a result, your bones become weak and break easily. Good sources are milk, cheese, yogurt, beans, soybeans, spinach, and figs.

Copper

Copper is involved in the absorption, storage, and metabolism of iron and in the formation of red blood cells. It also helps supply oxygen to the body. The symptoms of copper deficiency are similar to iron-deficiency anemia. Kiwi and lima beans have a significant amount of copper, as do legumes, molasses, prunes, seafood, soybeans, apples, bananas, and blackberries.

Chromium

Chromium maintains blood sugar levels, helps sugar metabolize, helps burn fat, lowers high blood pressure, and helps people lose weight. Lack of chromium increases the likelihood of diabetes, hypoglycemia, high cholesterol, and hypertension.

Sources include meat, molasses, rice bran, shellfish, and wheat germ.

Iodine

Iodine helps regulate the rate of energy production and body weight and promotes proper growth. Iodine reduces body fat, relieves anxiety and nervousness, increases energy, helps skin and hair, and boosts the immune system. It also promotes healthy hair, nails, skin, and teeth. In countries where iodine is deficient in the soil, rates of hypothyroidism, goiter, and retarded growth are very high. In developed countries, however, iodine is added to table salt and iodine deficiencies are rare. Sources are iodized salt, onions, tuna, and seaweed.

Iron

Iron deficiency in infants can result in impaired learning ability and behavioral problems. It affects the immune system and causes weakness and fatigue. To aid in the absorption of iron, eat foods rich in vitamin C at the same time you eat the food containing iron. Take iron supplements and your vitamin E at different times of the day, as iron supplements tend to neutralize the vitamin E. Vegetarians need to get twice as much dietary iron as meat eaters. Probably the best sources of iron for all ages are raisins and blackberries.

Magnesium

Magnesium is needed for building strong bone cells, protein, making new cells, activating B vitamins, relaxing nerves and muscles, clotting blood, secreting insulin, and maintaining energy. Magnesium also assists in the absorption of calcium, vitamin C, and potassium. Deficiency may result in fatigue, nervousness, insomnia, heart problems, high blood pressure, osteoporosis, muscle weakness, and cramps. Large quantities of magnesium are contained in kiwi, bananas, and nuts.

Manganese

Manganese functions in enzyme reactions concerning blood sugar, metabolism, and thyroid hormone function. It's an activator for cartilage and bone development. Manganese deficiency can lead to deafness, asthma, carpal tunnel syndrome, and birth defects. Most fruits contain manganese, with blackberries and strawberries having significant amounts. Peas, lima beans, sweet potatoes, and nuts are also excellent sources.

Phosphorous

In combination with calcium, phosphorus is necessary for the formation of bones, teeth, and nerve cells. It is widely distributed in other plant and animal foods, so it's unlikely that deficiency would be a problem.

Potassium

Without this mineral, you will feel like something the cat drug in. You will feel too exhausted and weak to climb stairs and too tired to breathe. Your muscles will cramp, and your heart rhythms will be erratic and disturbed. Potassium is essential for the body's growth and maintenance and to keep a normal water balance between cells and body fluids. It plays an essential role in proper heart function. Deficiency may cause muscular cramps, twitching, weakness, irregular heartbeat, insomnia, and kidney and lung failure. Potassium is found in most fruits, vegetables, and nuts.

Selenium

Generally selenium functions as an antioxidant that works in conjunction with vitamin E to prevent cancers, increase immune response, protect against heart disease, boost energy and sex drive, and help protect against arthritis and multiple sclerosis. It is found in nuts, onions, tuna, and wheat germ, as well as most fruits and vegetables.

Sodium

Sodium is required by the body to regulate blood pressure and blood volume. It helps regulate the fluid balance in your body. Sodium also assists in the proper functioning of muscles and nerves. Sodium occurs naturally in almost all nuts and fresh, whole fruits and vegetables.

Zinc

Zinc is essential for protein and carbohydrate metabolism to the immune system, wound healing, growth, and vision. Severe deficiency can contribute to stunted growth and can sometimes be seen in white spots on the fingernails. Zinc is used to treat arthritis, boils, skin ulcers, acne, peptic ulcers, and enlarged prostate. It is found in beef, dark poultry meat (legs, thighs, and wings), fish, organ meats, pumpkin and squash seeds, wheat germ, and yogurt.

Chapter 5

Processed Sugars

"A little poison is still poison."

IF YOU WANT TO be free of sugar cravings, eat as little sugar as possible. Processed sugars add no nutrition to your body and fuel your appetite by causing you to become ravenously hungry within minutes after eating. It drives your cravings.

After being off sugar for a year, I was rather astonished to find that occasionally I could skip either lunch or dinner entirely and not bother to snack until the next meal. When sugar isn't driving your appetite and reminding you that you need food every minute, you can actually accomplish more and live on much less. One slice of cheese or one raw fruit serving is now enough to dull my appetite and forget about eating for hours. I would not have believed this was possible in my last life (before a no-sugar lifestyle).

Sugar Content

Look at the sugar content in fruit-flavored yogurt, fruit bars, and supposedly other "health" foods. Note the extensive list of food dyes and chemical additives. Sugar can now be disguised under dozens of different names, such as sucrose, fructose, corn syrup, malt, cane syrup, and so on.

So-called diet or health snack bars are designed to sell

by stamping the names of popular diets or buzzwords (e.g., "Zone," "High Protein," or "Low-Carb") somewhere on the package. If you scan their ingredients, you will find that they are anything but healthy, and definitely will not help you lose weight. They are high in sugar, loaded with unhealthy simple carbs and little nutrition. Some may even insist that they are low-carb, but 20 grams of sugar amounts to about 5 teaspoons. There doesn't seem to be any guidelines as to what these manufacturers can label "low-carb." Excuse me, but 5 teaspoons of sugar in anything is not low-carb! If sugar or one of its disguised substitutes (corn syrup, sucrose, fructose, malt, and so on) is the first ingredient on the list, this means there is more sugar in that product than any other ingredient listed after it. If it's second on the list, only the first item listed is more prevalent in that product. **Sugar is the substance that makes you hungry and keeps your appetite running at full blast.** Some products may have three or more different sugars.

I happen to enjoy raisin bran (the no-sugar variety from a health-food store) all by itself for breakfast. I have consumed it for years without adding sugar or milk. I pour myself a bowlful of dry flakes and eat it along with a glass of orange juice or plain, unsweetened green tea. I don't use normal milk because of lactose intolerance and have never developed a taste for soy or rice milk. Sugarless raisin bran doesn't trigger my sugar cravings, and provides me with necessary fiber. If I were to sprinkle sugar on top by one or more spoonfuls, it would make it entirely unhealthy by raising my insulin levels considerably. By midmorning I would be so hungry, I'd eat numerous calories before lunchtime.

If you buy supposed healthier cereals in a normal mega-supermarket, you will note that some have up to three or four different processed sugars within the first five or six ingredients. They may have brown sugar, cane sugar, malt sugar, fructose, corn syrup, or by any other disguised name all in the same package. These are not healthy foods, and consuming them will make it very difficult, if not impossible, for you to lose weight.

After my weight stabilized at 160 pounds for two months, I looked closely at the sugar content of the remaining foods I was eating. Even though my source of raisin bran from the normal supermarket was lower in sugar than most cereals, it still contained an astonishing 20 percent. For every five spoonfuls of cereal, I was eating at least one spoonful of processed sugar. My brand of peanut butter was also high in sugar and hydrogenated oil. I discontinued using both. I switched to a type of raisin bran with no processed sugar at all and went back to old-fashioned peanut butter that doesn't clog arteries. Some brands of old-fashioned peanut butter already come premixed with honey, which is also acceptable as long as processed sugar isn't hiding in those ingredients. After these minor changes, taking care not to eat if I was not hungry, and picking up some extra workouts, the weight began to drop again.

One breakfast meal that is disastrous for diabetics or those of us who are sugar addicts is pancakes, waffles, or French toast dripping with syrup. Syrup has over ten teaspoons of sugar per one-fourth cup serving or the equivalent of just a little over three tablespoons of sugar to make up that quarter cup. Remember that one-fourth cup of liquid is equivalent to only four tablespoons. Try pancakes with unsweetened applesauce instead. You will have to check carefully to find applesauce that does not contain any sweeteners. This is incredibly filling, delicious, and doesn't trigger your blood sugars to launch you into a coma. Since pancakes are pure starch, you will need to limit the serving size and how often you eat them.

Another high-fiber breakfast food is whole-grain, heavy bread (found at the nearest health-food shop). Toast yourself a slice and spread with unsweetened cream cheese or peanut butter. This should satisfy you for hours.

Remember when lemonade was made from real lemons? The lemonade that is packaged today is oversweetened and dyed to the unappetizing color of urine. I never touch sweetened drinks anymore because of my sugar addiction, but before my new life I used to add just a quick squirt of lemonade from the fast-food drink machine to my unsweetened iced tea. When I was a child, lemonade used to be sweetened with only a pinch of sugar, barely enough to taste the sweetness—just enough to dull the sour taste of the lemons. I think lemonade manufacturers today take a bag of sugar and add a touch of lemon.

When I made the commitment to boycott sugar, it was after growing concern that I was becoming diabetic. My insulin levels were erratic from years of sugar abuse. If I went without eating for more than two or three hours during the day, I would become light-headed and irritable and would need to eat something to physically feel better. Sometimes, I noticed slight shaking in my hands if I let myself go too long without eating. I was especially vulnerable during extremely hot weather where my energy level would dip and I could not seem to replace fluid quickly enough.

I was a sugar-holic, especially where chocolate was concerned. I could not keep ice cream or cookies in my house because I would nibble at them until the package was empty. I would keep forking a pie or cake until the entire dessert was consumed. To keep myself from having those temptations immediately available, I banned desserts from my home years ago. Eating that amount of "poison" at one sitting can kill you slowly over time by depleting your health.

To prevent this disaster, I stopped purchasing the larger containers and bought pint-sized milk chocolate ice cream or the tiny, expensive packages that contained only two chocolate chip cookies. That would satisfy me temporarily. The rich, pint-size, creamy chocolate ice creams that I enjoyed contained 1,200 calories. I would eat the entire pint in one sitting in the grocery store parking lot. At that time I always carried an unbendable metal spoon in my purse for such occasions. Since then, I've trashed the spoon because I don't eat frozen ice cream anymore—or any desserts anymore for that matter. It's a wonder that I didn't exceed half a ton, but I know that only my consistent exercise routines spared me from total disaster.

If I made a batch of chocolate chip cookie dough for kids' events at school, I would consume all the dough before I could get it into the oven. Therefore, I automatically doubled or tripled the recipe each time to allow enough to eat raw and the rest for baking. Later, I learned to buy prepackaged cookies for school events in flavors that didn't tempt me. Years ago, I stopped making cookies and stopped bringing them home. For an outrageous sum of money, I would buy only one cookie at a specialty cookie counter where individual cookies were sold. I stopped making desserts for the holidays. I knew that if I made them, I would eat them. They were not good for me, so why should I make them for the grandkids? The grandkids received enough junk food over the holidays without my adding to the pile. I had to convince myself that my grandchildren would not be deprived without my offering them unhealthy foods at the holidays. I had to give myself permission that it was okay not to give my grandchildren these "treats." If it was harmful to my health, it would also be harmful to theirs. They get enough junk treats in school and at parties, where it's beyond my control. Good memories could still be passed on to the children that do not relate to sweet, unhealthy foods around the holidays.

Once I worked through this mental cycle, addictive foods had less of a hold because I did not allow their presence in my home. I gave my grandchildren small nonfood, noncandy treats for holidays or their birthdays that did not include trash foods. The sugar industry has made it too easy for us to overindulge ourselves in these products. It is customary to have chocolates at Easter, candies on Valentine's Day and Halloween, cake for birthdays, pie for Thanksgiving, goodies galore at Christmas, and so on. Children get so much unnecessary sweets and chocolate in their classrooms around the holidays that they certainly don't need more from you.

Sticky Sugar

Sugar is sticky. When sugar attaches to collagen proteins in your body, clumps form. This means that your blood vessels, lungs, and joints all stiffen and your skin sags. They cloud the proteins in the lens of your eye, causing cataracts. They affect production of more than fifty thousand different proteins your body makes to regulate its functions. They tend to form in clumps very similar to the tangles and plaques that are found in the brains of Alzheimer's patients.

Our Sugar Consumption

In 1900, people consumed only a few teaspoons of sugar per day, much of which included real honey, which is loaded with natural enzymes. Also used was a heavy form of molasses that contained iron and numerous other natural vitamins and minerals.

The USDA currently recommends that the average person eat no more than ten teaspoons of sugar per day, but the average American in 2005 ate fifty-three teaspoons of sugar each day, or 212 grams. **One teaspoon of sugar is equivalent to four grams.** Fifty-three teaspoons of sugar is equal to over 1 cup of sugar per day per every man, woman, and child in this country. If sugar were a nourishing healthful substance, then no harm done. If processed sugar creates an atmosphere for disease to grow in your body as well as cause the harmful side effects of obesity, which it does indeed do, then we need to drastically alter our eating patterns — NOW!

Hold the Sugar

Imagine pouring a five-pound bag of sugar down your child's throat. This is the amount kids get **every month**, and most of it doesn't come from the sugar bowl or cookie jar. Liquid sugar from soda, sweetened juice, and fruit drinks is the biggest source.

Too much of any sweetener (dextrose, cane juice, fructose, fruit juice concentrate, glucose, high-fructose corn syrup, honey, lactose, maple syrup, molasses, sucrose) can raise a child's risk of obesity, cause poor bone density, and result in type two diabetes by adding calories and crowding out healthier dairy products, fruits, and vegetables. Sweetener overload also contributes to tooth decay and spoils a child's taste for real foods.

Fun-filled ads that push candy, sugar-filled cereals, fruit drinks, and sodas onto kids are geared toward getting them hooked early and making them customers for life.

Hidden in thousands of everyday foods is an insidious source of empty calories that make a beeline for your belly, butt, and thighs: sugars (including high-fructose corn syrup, the major processed-food sweetener). These sugars are added to enhance the flavors of many processed foods, so we eat more of them. Even foods you'd never expect—for example, French fries and certain potato chips and crackers—are sweetened.

Not only does sugar make you fat and decay your teeth, but that may be the least of it. It also causes your pancreas to go into overdrive, pumping out insulin as a way of balancing the sugar in your bloodstream.

Yeast Infections

A source of toxins in your body could very well be your own digestive system. If you can't eliminate toxins well, your overall health will suffer and any health problems you do have will be accentuated if the intestinal tract accumulates toxic waste products. Of even more concern are toxins created in your intestinal tract by the presence of a yeast overgrowth, also known as candidiasis. This problem has achieved epidemic proportions.

Ordinarily, your intestines contain trillions of bacteria that are essential to your digestion. They are a vital part of the process that breaks down your food into nutrients you can absorb.

Often, however, those beneficial bacteria get crowded out by an overgrowth of the yeastlike organism called Candida albicans, which is a normal resident of the large intestine. A host of medical and dietary abuses can cause this to happen. The major cause is the use of antibiotics, which kill off the beneficial bacteria that otherwise hold the growth of the yeast in check. Yeast also overgrows from the use of hormones such as prednisone, body-building steroids, and birth-control pills.

Another culprit is too much sugar in the diet, followed closely by foods that are high in natural sugar, such as fruit, honey, fruit juice, and milk. Alcohol, food additives, food intolerances (especially lactose or gluten intolerance), insufficient stomach acid, and emotional stress can all trigger yeast overgrowth.

Yeast overgrowth is often a key ingredient in the larger disease picture of conditions such as chronic fatigue syndrome, frequently recurring infections, Crohn's disease, colitis, and irritable bowel syndrome. It's also a major contributor to food intolerances. The yeast diagnosis can be inferred by a variety of symptoms, especially lower intestinal gas and bloating, frequent bouts of diarrhea and constipation, decreased resistance to infection, chronic fatigue syndrome, "brain fog," recurrent bladder infections, and thrush, a whitish plaque in the mouth and throat. Joint pain, fatigue, and depression are also common symptoms. Yeast overgrowth is also strongly associated with arthritis.

Yeast in your intestines lives on sugar, so the first step in curing an overgrowth is simply to deprive yeast of its favorite food. Those of you with yeast infections should switch to a low-carbohydrate, sugar-free diet (skip the artificial sugars, too) that eliminates all simple sugars as well as all cured, salted, fermented, or yeast-containing foods, such as cheese, vinegar, alcohol, and bread.

Sugar-Free and Low-Sugar Foods Can Cause Gas, Cramps, and Diarrhea

Instead of sugar, these products use sugar alcohols: maltitol, sorbitol, xylitol, mannitol, lactitol, and erythritol. Inside your body, sugar alcohols are digested by intestinal bacteria instead of sugar-digesting enzymes. Limiting these products reduces your gas, cramps, and diarrhea.

High-Fructose Corn Syrup

High-fructose corn syrup (HFCS) is relatively cheap and easy to use (thanks to its syrup form). It now accounts for almost half of all caloric sweeteners added to foods and beverages.

One possible link between HFCS, obesity, and type two diabetes is the way our bodies process fructose. Normally, eating sweet foods stimulates insulin, a hormone that converts sugar to glucose (the form of sugar that cells burn for energy). As your body's energy needs are met, insulin triggers fullness. The problem with fructose is that it doesn't stimulate insulin to the same degree that other sugars do, which means that the body doesn't release the hormone leptin. Our bodies don't know when we are full.

The more fructose in a meal, the less insulin you'll secrete. Heart disease is also a potential concern. When sugar bypasses insulin, it's converted to fat. Fructose also seems to drive up the levels of blood fats, a risk factor for heart disease.

By skipping foods with HFCS, you will avoid other added sugars listed on labels under names such as fruit juice concentrate, evaporated cane juice, malt, sucrose, fructose, and caramel. Sugar, no matter what name it goes by, is still calories with no nutritional value. You'll find HFCS in items from ketchup and pasta sauce to English muffins, cereal, and yogurt. We get about two-thirds of it from sweetened beverages such as sodas, iced tea, lemonade, and fruit drinks.

In our generation, one of the largest changes in our diet has been the increase in the use of high-fructose corn syrup. Use of this substance has risen to most of the sugar consumption per person per year. Fructose is processed more rapidly and efficiently than glucose, therefore, **we have ingested what can be viewed as fat for fat storage!**

Larger Plates Make Larger Bodies

When we entered the supersize era, the food purveyors noticed that people would not purchase two small bags of French fries—because of the possible fear of being thought gluttonous—but had no problem buying one huge bag of the same product. This led to supersized meals of all kinds. The size of serving plates in restaurants has typically increased. Since the number of calories obtained away from home keeps rising, there is increased exposure to greater amounts of food. We don't have to eat it all—but we do.

In my past state of obesity, I wouldn't leave food on my plate uneaten. It was an obsession to clean my plate, and I did. It went straight to the fat storage section of my body.

Today, without the sugar addiction driving compulsive hunger, I no longer have any qualms regarding leftover food on my plate. I also have three dogs who will eat anything, so nothing goes to waste, or to *my* waist.

No Soda, Please

We all know that soft drinks are a good habit to break. Here are some surprising new motivators: Women drinking more than one sugared soda daily doubled their chances of getting type two diabetes.

Sugar-filled soda really does rot teeth. Malic and tartaric acids in sodas damage dental enamel. Caffeine, carbonation, and sugar substitutes can irritate your bladder, keeping you running to the bathroom.

To help you get an idea of how much sugar is in our popular foods, please note the following chart:

Sugar Content of Popular Foods (1 teaspoon of sugar is equal to 4 grams)

Food	Sugar Contents in Teaspoons
Cola, 12 ounces	9 ½
Vanilla yogurt, 8 ounces	2 ½
Yogurt with fruit on the bottom, 8 ounces	9
Yogurt, low-fat, fruit-flavored, 8 ounces	7
Snickers bar, 2.1 ounces	5 ¾
TastyKake Honey Bun, 3 ¼ ounces	6
Entenmann's Chocolate Fudge Cake, 3 ounces	8 ½
Burger King Cini-minis w/icing, 4.7 ounces	9 ½
Pepsi, 12 ounces	10 ¼
Pancake syrup, ¼ cup	10 ¼
Hostess Lemon Fruit Pie, 4 ½ ounces	11 ½
McDonald's Vanilla Shake, 20 ounces	12
Cinnabon, 7 ½ ounces	12 ¼
Sunkist Orange Soda, 12 ounces	13
McDonald's McFlurry w/ Butterfingers, 10 ounces	13 ¾
Strawberry Passion Awareness Fruitopia, 20 ounces	17 ¾
Dairy Queen Mr. Misty Slush, 32 ounces	28

This chart should open your eyes to how much sugar you are consuming. The FDA only offers a recommended daily amount of ten teaspoons of sugar. You don't have to eat that much or any at all. **Sugar has no nutritional value**, so less is better and none at all gives your body a chance to eat more of substances that may actually be good for you. It's virtually impossible to eat completely sugar-free foods in our country because sugar is hidden in almost every item of prepackaged food. (And don't substitute sugar-free chemicals in place of sugar because those are even worse for your health.) It's added to ketchup, BBQ sauce, soups, crackers, and other foods that you would not normally think of as needing sugar. If you think crackers are sugar-free, look again. That may be why you can't eat just one.

If anything chocolate was served at an event, I used to help myself to as much as my plate would hold and go back for more. If I did not satisfy my chocolate fix each day, I developed a light "caffeine headache."

We are the first generation to be snowed under with this sugar assault. It's taken a generation passing before the results of this sugar avalanche could be studied and understood how it relates to insulin levels and obesity. I knew that eating too much sugar was making me fat, but I didn't understand how to stop my addiction in its tracks.

I cannot remember a time in my "fat life" when I did not crave chocolate. I would plan my day around chocolate and when and where I could get my next "fix." I used chocolate sweets to satiate my hunger and alleviate any stress.

I remember once having a discussion with my daughter about my eating behavior as if this were normal, and she gave me such a strange look as if to say "You think this is normal, Mom?" It was at that moment I fully realized the extent of my sugar addiction. We both laugh at that incident now, but it was the beginning of my new reality.

Insulin

Insulin is sometimes referred to as the hunger hormone because it stimulates people to eat. When insulin is released in normal people minutes after they start eating, it may cause them to feel hungrier than they thought they were when they started eating. But upon completing their meal they feel satisfied; their insulin level drops and their brains get the signal to stop eating.

Hours later, after the body has used some of the glucose, the insulin-to-glucose ratio in blood changes. It appears that this rise signals the body to eat again. We recognize this signal as the sensation of hunger. The normal person then eats, and the whole process begins again.

The balance of carbohydrates and insulin is a delicate one—and it can malfunction. Within a few minutes of eating simple carbohydrates (those foods with processed sugars), the carbohydrate addict's body releases far more insulin than is necessary. This overabundance of insulin "insults" the cells that should be taking up the carbohydrate energy (glucose), interfering with the normal absorption of glucose.

An excess of insulin remains in the bloodstream. As insulin levels fail to drop, the brain levels of the chemical serotonin fail to rise and the carbohydrate addict may not feel satisfied. Some carbohydrate addicts state that they do feel satisfied after eating, others that they find they again feel like eating within two hours or so. And if the carbohydrate addict attempts to satisfy his or her hunger by again consuming carbohydrates, the insulin release that follows will be even greater and the sense of satisfaction even less. All of the above was true in my sugar addiction.

Many carbohydrate addicts report that their cravings grow stronger each time they eat carbohydrates. They find themselves in a continuous cycle of eating, craving, and eating again.

In the presence of excess insulin, the body also becomes very good at conserving energy. **So while the carbohydrate addict gets hungrier after each carbohydrate-rich meal, the body gets better at storing energy—in the form of fat.**

Subconscious hunger is characterized by a strong and often uncontrollable desire to eat; it results in the consumption of food without plan or anticipation. Carbohydrate addicts often have an **impulse-eating** incident with little awareness. Normal eaters and lower-level carbohydrate addicts attribute the impulse-eating incidents to habit, though occasionally they admit that they are unable to stop even when they want to. **During impulse eating, food is often consumed quickly with little** chewing and with almost gulping reflexes or shoveling it down. Addictive types of food cause this stuffing or overeating "reflex."

Serotonin levels don't rise sufficiently to cause satisfaction; the carbohydrate addict does not get the signal to stop eating and continues to eat carbohydrate-rich foods. **Greater and more frequent quantities of carbohydrates may be consumed with no increase in satisfaction.**

When a carbohydrate addict eats carbohydrates, his or her body releases too much of the "hunger hormone," insulin, into the bloodstream. Rather than telling the brain that hunger has been satisfied, this excess of insulin (hyperinsulinemia) causes the carbohydrate addict to desire more food after eating. **Carbohydrate addicts often feel driven to eat.** Yet **the more often sweets, starches, and snack foods are eaten, the more insulin is produced and the more frequent and stronger are the cravings for carbohydrate-rich foods.**

Because of the way carbohydrate addicts react to certain foods they eat (i.e., because of their metabolism), **most carbohydrate addicts experience hunger or recurring cravings much more intensely and more often than do normal people, and the only way they can feel better physically is to eat.** They may feel a sense of irritation, anxiety, or anger. And these responses seem to get stronger over time.

Consuming high-carbohydrate foods is another surefire way to trigger the desire for more carbohydrates. Among the foods that most dieters find trigger their addictions are:

- Bread and other grain products, including bagels, cookies, cereals, cakes, crackers, pastries, donuts, and rolls.

- Sweet dessert foods, including ice cream, chocolate, candy, puddings, sherbets, cakes, sweet rolls, cookies, sweet drinks, or anything else sweetened with refined sugars.

- Snack foods like popcorn, potato chips, pretzels, cheese puffs, and nuts.

- And other foods, too, including some beans (Boston baked beans, rich with molasses, is a classic trigger); all kinds of pasta, from simple spaghetti and egg noodles to ravioli; rice (alone and in other dishes); French fries; and plain sugar, even just a spoonful in your coffee or tea.

When carbohydrates are eaten less frequently, less insulin is produced. The body has a lowered tendency to store the excess calories in its fat cells and is more capable of breaking down stored fat. The less often the carbohydrate addict consumes sugary foods, the more satisfying the foods are and the greater the control of eating that is possible. **The overweight carbohydrate-addiction cycle can be broken by removing processed sugar from your diet.**

Less sugar means less insulin, which means less hunger, fewer cravings, and a feeling of satisfaction. Best of all, a lowered level of insulin prods your body to take fat out of storage and use it.

If our blood sugar stays too high for long, we develop a host of problems in short order: blurred vision, excessive urination, thirst, dehydration, dizziness, coma, and even death. Excess insulin circulating throughout the body causes heart disease, diabetes, elevated cholesterol and triglycerides, high blood pressure, and other disease misery we modern humans suffer as we age.

The average person can actually reverse an insulin-related disorder by switching to a healthier diet.

Excess insulin, largely the consequence of eating a diet that contains much more sugar and starch (unlike our ancestors ate seventy-five or more years ago), sets the stage for development of insulin resistance and type two diabetes. Given our modern taste for carbo junk—cookies, candies, cakes, ice cream, pies, muffins, donuts, bagels, breads, pasta, rolls, sugar-sweetened cereals, French fries—and the insulin rise such foods cause, it should come as no surprise that the incidence of type two diabetes has skyrocketed in the last thirty years. Amazingly, the standard treatment for type two diabetes in the last several decades has been the high-carbohydrate, low-fat diet. Fat was seen as the enemy of diabetics and a high-carbohydrate diet (which really means a diet high in sugar) as the remedy. Thankfully, for the sake of diabetic sufferers everywhere, the tide has begun to take a sensible turn toward a diet of lean protein, fat in essential oils such as that found in nuts or fish, and fewer simple carbohydrates (desserts and sweets).

Each time an insulin-resistant person eats a high-sugar, high-starch, insulin-raising meal, they're buying a one-way ticket for excess calories of any kind to be moved into their fat cells.

If we examine all the possible strategies to reduce insulin and improve insulin sensitivity to see where we can get the most bang for our buck in terms of insulin-lowering, we need to look no further than *restricting simple carbohydrates (all the sugary junk foods).*

If insulin levels are low enough, then fat storage pretty much shuts down.

The largest contributors of calories are soda, white bread, rolls, crackers, donuts, cookies, and cakes—i.e., junk. That's pitiful. It's no wonder there is so much obesity, heart disease, type two diabetes, and all the rest. As you might imagine, this horrendous dietary change has come at an enormous health cost.

By simply changing the way you eat to a diet lower in starch and sugar and higher in good-quality fats, you can reduce high cholesterol, lower your triglycerides, and reduce your risk for heart disease—without resorting to expensive and potentially damaging medications.

Sugar has a severely depressing effect on your immune system. Eating sweet foods of any sort interferes with the ability of your white blood cells to attack and destroy invading pathogens. The negative effect of just one glass of soda lowers your body's ability to produce antibodies. Are you always finishing up one cold or flu to begin another?

Get Real with What to Eat

To lose weight more rapidly, limit your **carbohydrate-rich,** high-glycemic foods, such as fruit, bread, or mashed potatoes, to no more than two to three servings per day. Merely removing desserts and sweets from your diet may not allow you to lose weight, or you may lose so slowly that you become discouraged if you continue to eat large quantities of bread, potatoes, pasta, or fruit. Eat these foods in limited quantities. You may even want to keep a journal for a few weeks to keep track of all the foods you are eating and which ones cause you to overeat. You might find that you are eating pastas or breads multiple times per day in the form of cereal, bagels, pizzas, rolls, or pasta. If any of these foods trigger your eating frenzy, remove them from your diet entirely or try limiting the servings of all the heavier carbs (those with higher glycemic levels). If you must have your French fries daily or bread with every meal, then you are sabotaging yourself and you will not succeed in losing weight. You will defeat your own purpose. Limit these foods to occasional occurrences.

At this point in my life, I have a metabolism that can handle large quantities of whole fruits and still maintain my weight. Some days I consume a fruit shake containing at least five servings of fruit, plus I eat two other whole fruits during the day. However, I tend to eat less of other foods on those days, so fruit is a large source of nourishment and calories during the season when my favorite fruits are available. The sweetness of fruit does not cause me to overeat, but it is a problem for some people, especially diabetics.

If you have diabetic tendencies, you may find that eating a whole fruit between meals triggers your eating mechanism or raises your blood sugar levels too high. If this happens, only eat fruit with meals that contain protein and no more than two servings of fruit per day, if your doctor says that is okay for you.

I've found that a spoonful of healthy peanut butter or slice of cheese works well to dull my hunger between meals. Peanut butter and cheese are both high in protein and essential oils and are extremely nutritious. Be careful of the peanut butter brands that are loaded with sugar and hydrogenated oil. I opt instead for a brand that is mixed only with honey and salt. Try eating servings of protein, such as scrambled eggs, along with your fruit serving for breakfast and see if that helps. A diet too low in protein will also cause your hunger levels to rise out of control.

Avoid high-sugar cereals. If you are serious about losing weight, you must delete them from your menu. Read their ingredient list. If sugar, fructose, malt, corn syrup, or any other "use" or "sugar cousin" is listed in the top five ingredients, you don't need it. To continue eating this product on a daily basis is only going to stop you from losing weight by keeping your hunger switch on. Switch to an unsweetened bagel (if it tastes sweet, there is too much sugar in your choice) with unsweetened cream cheese or scrambled eggs or an omelet for breakfast with a half cup of 100 percent juice or whole fruit. You don't need a twenty-ounce glass of fruit juice. This contains no fiber and may cause a reaction of flooding your body with insulin, which adds storage of fatty deposits. Eating the fruit in its natural state with all of its fiber slows down the insulin rush. Adding protein to your breakfast will leave you less hungry, and lunchtime will come without you even missing that snack between meals. For some people, your bread sensitivity might raise your insulin levels so high that you may need to avoid bagels. Try getting a heavier, grainier, health-food store variety that you can toast for extra flavor. Heavier, grainier breads are filling and keep your blood sugar from spiking.

Lunch can be satisfying with as much as you want to eat of a chunky style soup and/or salad or a main dish served with plenty of green or yellow vegetables. For dinner, eat as much as you want of two vegetables and a main protein dish. Limit your serving size of potatoes or other starchy vegetables, especially for the evening meal, as they will slow your ability to lose weight. Your metabolism slows down while you are sleeping, so immediately available calories are more likely to travel into the fat storage areas of your body. Use lower-carb vegetables that you enjoy in the evening and eat as much as you want.

Try to eat dinner early in the evening so that you have time to burn calories before bedtime. It also helps reduce restless sleep patterns and nightmares if your stomach is not stuffed when you sleep.

When I accidentally order foods that have a highly sweetened sauce on the meat or vegetables, it repels me. My taste buds find it distasteful and repulsive. I don't need or want my meat and vegetables sweetened. Our society has gone sugar crazy. There is no sense in sweetening meats and vegetables. Our manufacturers even add sugar to naturally sweet fruit that is canned or juiced. This is further eroding health and our natural sense of taste. After you cut sugar from your way of life, you will notice when anything tastes sweet, and it becomes a turnoff.

Three Hours Before Bedtime

Many weight loss programs encourage you not to eat three hours before bedtime. If this is your time of grazing and snacking, *you may find this to be your greatest key to weight loss.* I've found this trick works especially well for me because I arrive home by 5:00 PM, and I'm in bed before 9:00 PM. As soon as I arrive home, I eat dinner and only drink water after that. It stopped **all** of my evening munching and excess calories. Improving your health starts by changing one bad habit at a time. For me, evening snacking was a very bad habit!

Artificial Killers (Sweeteners)

For many years saccharin was widely used as an artificial sweetener, despite the fact that it can cause cancer in humans. After several attempts to ban the substance, the FDA finally removed it from the market in 1987.

Aspartame (NutraSweet, Equal) is the new favorite; it's a "natural" sweetener made of phenylalanine and aspartic acid, containing "nothing artificial." In the body, these naturally occurring substances break down into the same amino acids found in any protein food. Sounds harmless, but it isn't. I even found this substance in my chewable vitamin C, which I immediately trashed and found another brand that wasn't detrimental to my health.

The problem with aspartame is that **large doses of phenylalanine are toxic to the brain and can cause mental retardation and seizures in people with phenylkeonuria (PKU), a genetic disorder**. For others, the sweetener may cause chemical changes in the brain that contribute to headaches, depression, mood swings, high blood pressure, insomnia, **seizures,** and behavior problems. It can also cause your appetite control center to malfunction, so your diet drinks may be causing more harm than good. Aspartame may also cause birth defects, such as mild retardation, and is not recommended for use by pregnant women.

Because aspartame is found in so many products, it is very easy to overdose without realizing it. When you take a vitamin pill with aspartame, eat your breakfast cereal and hot cocoa with aspartame, have some aspartame-sweetened gelatin and a soft drink for lunch, chocolate pudding with aspartame for dinner dessert, and maybe another soda, it adds up very quickly. Children could easily consume twice the FDA limit every day and possibly suffer learning impairment and behavior problems. **Part of the problem with the current labeling of aspartame is that the actual amounts used do not have to be**

listed, so you really have no idea how much aspartame you are consuming. Remember, the FDA only recommends a daily amount that won't kill you immediately, but no aspartame is healthy.

Learn to develop a taste for foods that are not sweet.

Aspartame is used primarily to make our foods low in calories and low in sugars. Used heavily by the diet industry, aspartame is made up of three chemicals: aspartic acid, phenylalanine, and methanol.

- *Aspartic Acid:* Causes lesions in the brains of lab animals and changes their DNA. This means that future generations can be affected, producing obese and sexually dysfunctional lab animals (and we don't know all the terrible affects it has on humans).

- *Phenylalanine:* This chemical can cause seizures and brain tumors. Is it just coincidence that brain tumors are on the rise?

- *Methanol:* Causes depression. In fluid form, methanol (wood alcohol) breaks down into formic acid (used in industry to strip epoxy and urethane coatings) and formaldehyde (used for embalming corpses). In other words, it is killing you.

If you think our government would ban a substance this toxic, they might, but only after serious years of fighting between the lobbyists and special interest groups. In the meantime, your health is at stake. Don't risk it.

Aspartame consumption has been connected with headaches, joint pain, memory loss, numbness, tinnitus, hearing loss, vision problems, weight gain, rashes, seizures, fatigue, muscle spasms, dizziness, asthma, and chest tightness. Are you having any of these symptoms? Cut out the artificial sweeteners now! **Waiting to stop your dependency on these terrible** sweeteners unless you have symptoms may already be doing irreparable harm to your body.

Many people diagnosed with multiple sclerosis have lost all symptoms once they stopped using aspartame.

Aspartame can be hidden in anything: sugarless chewing gum, soft drinks, flavored water, drugs (prescription and over-the-counter), vitamin and herb supplements, yogurt, instant breakfasts, candy, breath mints, cereals, cocoa mixes, coffee beverages, gelatin desserts, frozen desserts, juice beverages, laxatives, fiber powders, milk drinks, shake mixes, tabletop sweeteners, tea beverages, instant teas and coffees, topping mixes, wine coolers, and so on.

Other sweeteners to avoid are NutriSweet, Equal, canderel, neotame, sucralose (Splenda), acesulfame-K (Sunette, Sweet & Safe, Sweet One), cyclamates, saccharin, refined sugar, and high-fructose sweeteners.

Honey Benefits

Until several hundred years ago, the only sweeteners used were honey, molasses, and fruit. When early explorers discovered sugar cane, they began to refine sugar. Because sugar is easier to store, easier to ship, doesn't harden, and doesn't spoil quickly, it pushed honey (with all its health benefits) to the back of the shelf.

Honey is **digested much more slowly** than regular table sugar. Honey is also loaded with nutrients: potassium, sulfur, sodium, phosphorus, magnesium, silica, copper, iron, manganese, enzymes, amino acids, B vitamins, vitamin C, and nucleic acids.

For thousands of years, honey was used as an antibacterial salve for wounds, sores, and skin ulcers. Honey stops bacteria by drawing water out of damaged tissue. Honey also helps healing by promoting cell growth on the edges of a cut and by working with the body's cells to generate an antiseptic. Honey has been used to stop even the nasty *Staphylococcus aureus* bacteria, a frequent cause of infection. We've forgotten about these earlier simple cures that our great-grandparents would not have survived without.

Honey has been used as a treatment for fevers, sore throats, insomnia, snake bites, and upset stomachs. It is also rich in antioxidants.

Honey is not recommended for infants, as their digestive systems are not fully developed enough to safely assimilate it.

Blackstrap Molasses

Blackstrap molasses has long been known to eliminate pain in the joints and was taken faithfully by my parents' generation. Unsulphured molasses is an excellent source of minerals, including iron, potassium, and magnesium. Blackstrap molasses is a great alternative to sweeten pancakes and hot cereal.

CHAPTER 6

Death and Life Are in Your Colon

"You only live once, but do you consider it living?"

A CORPSE IN OUR COUNTRY today takes longer to rot then it did one hundred years ago. Years of eating unnaturally processed, cooked, frozen, canned, irradiated, and chemically and genetically altered and preserved foods have contributed to the fact that undertakers will tell you that corpses rarely need to be embalmed these days; we unwittingly eat so many preservatives that our bodies now take much longer to decompose after death.

It is likely that many of you reading this have colons that are distorted and coated in stagnant, impacted feces. Just about everyone who eats western food does. Certainly, if you have a thick waistline or bulging abdomen, this is very likely to be the case.

Mucoid plaque forms in the colon as a defense mechanism against toxins. The mucus can be cleared away by pancreatic juices, but mucus-forming food now forms such a huge percentage of the western diet that the pancreas cannot cope.

Layers of plaque build up throughout the length of the intestinal tract and then compact and harden. A healthy colon contains residual friendly bacteria that can weigh up to five pounds; encrusted colons have been found at autopsies to

weigh forty pounds or more. Sometimes there is so much pu-
trid matter that parts of the colon expand from a normal two
and a half inches in diameter to an obscene ten or even twenty
inches wide in very obese people, leaving a channel of only
about a pencil's width in the center through which excreted
matter can pass. This leads to colon blockage and often lands
the misfortunate person in the hospital for surgery.

The colon becomes permanently toxic, and all manner of
health problems result as these poisons seep into your bloodstream and find their way to all parts of your body.

If you have ever consumed meat, poultry, fish, dairy products, sugar, processed foods, chocolate, caffeine, soft drinks, or
alcohol, then you will certainly have mucoid plaque and could
benefit from colon cleansing, which many herbalists advocate
as the cure for most diseases.

Constipation Is Unhealthy

Sometimes people are constipated and don't even know it.
They become so accustomed to feeling tired, bloated, irritated,
or overweight that they don't suspect their health is in danger.
Or they may be on medications to cover up such symptoms
and never seek the underlying cause.

If constipation is not addressed in time, it can slowly destroy a healthy body.

Serious Trouble Waiting to Happen

Having a bowel movement every two or three days is not suf-
ficient and definitely not healthy. A person with a healthy colon who is eating enough fruits, vegetables, and whole grains
should have at least two bowel movements per day. A healthy
body should be eliminating waste materials from every meal
you eat. Elimination should be complete, fast, and easy. The
stool should be light brown in color, long and large in diameter, and "fluffy" in texture. It should break apart with the
toilet flushing. Going to the bathroom once every few days,

sitting there straining for a half hour and passing black, hard "pebbles" that drop to the bottom is not only abnormal, but a warning that your body is in trouble. If you care about your health, pay attention.

If you are not eliminating approximately the same amount you are eating, then what do you think happens to the remainder of waste? The accumulation of old, hardened feces sticks to the colon walls, inhibiting its proper function of absorbing the remaining nutrients from the fecal matter. Instead, it is forced to absorb toxins from the buildup and from the parasites that make this debris their breeding ground. The passage through which the feces are forced to travel is also greatly reduced in diameter, so stools become much narrower—even as thin as a pencil sometimes. Common causes of constipation can be lack of fiber (whole grains, whole fruits, and vegetables) or not enough liquids in your diet; lack of exercise; medications that constipate; changes in life or routine such as pregnancy, older age, or travel; abuse of laxatives; or ignoring the urge to have a bowel movement (holding it in). Also, specific diseases such as a stroke can cause you to become constipated.

As long as the amount of toxin does not exceed the capacity of your excretory systems to eliminate it, health and vitality are easily maintained. However, sooner or later the toxic overload of daily life exceeds your body's ability to properly cleanse itself, and that's when toxemia develops and disease and degeneration begin.

Poor bowel movements are a big problem for most Americans these days. With long strands of mucus hanging around in your intestinal tract, stomach, and colon, it's easy to understand how ulcers, weight, and poor bowel movements mess with your energy and health.

Being blocked up with toxic waste helps explain why so many Americans have overweight issues, various cancers, heart disease, high blood pressure, skin problems, low energy, low immunity, and high incidences of flu, colds, and head-aches/migraines.

Less than one bowel movement per day, every day, is unacceptable and very unhealthy. An evacuation a day keeps the doctor away.

Constipation contributes to the lowering of the body's resistance, preparing the body for many acute illnesses, and begins many degenerative and chronic processes. The digestive system is the hub of the entire body. It feeds all our glands, organs, and every single cell. When the digestive system becomes sluggish, overly acidic, and toxic, it becomes less and less efficient. After the bowel becomes unnaturally acidic, it attempts to protect itself by secreting a glycoprotein substance that lines the entire intestinal wall—mucoid plaque.

Indeed, this condition can occur anywhere in the digestive tract where overacidity arises, including the esophagus, the stomach, the entire small intestine, and the colon.

Once this develops, proper digestion becomes more dysfunctional and constipation sets in. Then one problem occurs after another, and the bowel becomes a toxic sewer system. **Once the bowel becomes toxic, the blood becomes toxic, for all the blood coming from the bowel, carrying the necessary nutrients to feed the heart, lungs, brain, and muscles, goes to the liver—and nowhere else.** Then the liver must deal with the toxic blood. After years of relentless toxicity from the bowel, the liver becomes more sluggish. After a while it no longer functions efficiently, and toxic overloads begin to go to other parts of the body, such as the kidneys, heart, brain, joints, skin, lymph, and so on. Disease manifests where the toxins settle. When there is toxic settlement, there is lack of circulation, oxygen, and nutrients.

The very best of diets, the very best exercise routine, the very best herbal or dietary supplements, and the very best medications can be no better than the very worst if you're all clogged up inside, with a collection of chemical and toxic waste, ropes of mucus, and impacted feces accumulating and doing damage to your health and future health prospects.

Forget about the past. Now is the time to clean out your colon and move forward to better health.

No matter what your age, attaining and sustaining vigorous, energetic, youthful health demands that you focus equally on what goes into your body and what needs to come out of it. This is a continuous demand, not a one-time event. The more often you pay attention to this on a scheduled basis, the better off you will feel and look.

Cancer Connection and Colon Cleansing

Cancer is the final, fatal stage of tissue toxicity, but it takes a long time to develop. Long before it does, chronic toxemia takes its toll on human health in many other ways, making life miserable for millions of people who don't realize that the **root causes of their misery are their own blood and tissue toxicity from an overloaded colon.**

In addition to providing fertile ground for infection by germs, toxemia also damages the vital organs and impairs immune response, causing a wide range of degenerative ailments that grow steadily worse for as long as the state of toxicity continues.

Listed below are some of the most common symptoms associated with blood acidosis and tissue toxicity:

- Heartburn
- Allergies
- Headaches
- Festering sores
- Fungal infections
- Gastritis
- Psoriasis
- Sinusitus

- Fatigue
- Hair loss
- Arthritis
- Foul body odor
- Foul bad breath
- Frequent colds
- Vaginitis
- Depression
- Excess mucus
- Hyperactivity and anxiety
- All forms of cancer

While a variety of factors such as our American diet and harmful habits such as smoking or alcoholism may also be contributing causes in these conditions, the root cause always remains the same: toxemia.

Every cancer patient has this toxic waste lying around inside. No wonder cancer has a chance to take over the body, tissues, and cells.

The colon and lungs are considered paired organs in Chinese medicine. When the colon is afflicted with toxemia, the lungs are immediately afflicted too, and visa versa.

That's why doctors will tell you that there is such a strong correlation between colon cancer and lung cancer. With lung cancer present, colon cancer is almost always lurking in the background; likewise, where colon cancer is found, lung cancer is not far in the distance.

If you're a smoker and you want to avoid lung cancer, you must get this toxic mess out of your colon and continually be purifying your bloodstream before it starts burdening your lungs—ASAP. Once the colon collapses, the lungs are next.

If you are tired of asthma and allergies, now you know why it has never ended—even though you have taken tons of medications, drugs, and herbal products and used inhalers (which, by the way, are toxic and have steroids) for years. The colon-lung connection is where you need to take action.

An underactive colon full of toxic waste, combined with a polluted bloodstream and weak internal organs, invites disease in three ways, every day:

- It creates in itself a highly reactive, disease-friendly environment.

- Its slower transit time allows toxic substances to penetrate the bowel wall and pass into the blood and lymph where they spread throughout the body, creating greater vulnerability to disease in tissues already weakened by other means.

- When the amount of toxic material increases in the body from slowed bowels, the immune system goes haywire. The blood and lymph become polluted, and the only way to solve this problem includes colon cleansing and eating proper foods.

To eat whatever you want, anytime you want, and expect wonderful health, is irresponsible.

Within the colon and the folds of your colon lay five to forty pounds of smelly, foul, toxic impacted mucus.

One mistake most people make is to start using pharmaceutical drugs and surgical procedures to temporarily ease the discomfort and inconvenience of the chronic diseases and degenerative conditions caused by toxemia. That approach only makes the problems worse by increasing blood and tissue toxicity, while weakening immune response and other vital functions. The only effective way to deal with toxemia is to clean up your act with a regular program of bowel cleansing and a rational approach to eating healthy, nutritious, high-fiber foods daily.

Constipation and Your Liver and Gallbladder

Bile in your liver slows fermentation, oils the intestinal wall, prevents buildup of dangerous bacteria, stops tired intestinal epithelial cells, and stimulates the growth of new cells. **That's why it's so important not to overload the liver with pastries, foods rich in animal fat,** and so on. By transforming part of the bile and normalizing its flow, the gallbladder contributes to the detoxification function of the liver.

Eat whole wheat bread and high-fiber cereal, wheat and oat bran, fresh fruits and vegetables, figs and prunes (dried or fresh), and ground flaxseed. Flaxseed contains substances that lubricate the mucous membranes of the intestines, helping them eliminate waste products. Drink lots of water, and avoid the fiber supplements that contain sugar or artificial sugars. (Benefiber is an excellent choice; it mixes easily in any liquid, is tasteless, and doesn't solidify.)

Antibiotics, prescription drugs, and anesthetics can also mess up the proper flow of waste material from your bowels, as anyone who has recovered from surgery can testify. Also, major life changes such as pregnancy can cause extreme hormonal changes to the body that will impact your regularity. Large amounts of prunes and black figs will work to your advantage in most circumstances, regarding the usual compaction without resorting to laxatives.

How Do You Cleanse Your Colon?

I highly recommend Colonix as a thirty-to-ninety-day colon-cleansing product. This is a product that I have personally experienced, and it can be found at the website of www.drnatura.com. Colonix is gentle, it can be used while you do your normal activities, and it works. Many patients can testify that it also cleans out unusual parasites from their system. If you ever wondered what's down there, now is the time to find out.

"You cannot prevent the birds of sorrow from flying over your head, but you can prevent them from building nests in your hair."

—Chinese proverb

CHAPTER 7

Say It Out Loud

"What I say out loud is what I believe in my heart."

Your Speech Center Is in Control

THE SPEECH CENTER IN the brain exercises control over the whole central nervous system. You can actually cause different parts of the body to respond with stimuli to corresponding parts of the human brain, but when the speech center is stimulated, the whole central nervous system responds. Your body believes what your mouth speaks.

This means that when anyone says out loud, "I am an idiot," the speech center sends out the message to the whole body to prepare to be stupid.

"A word out of your mouth may seem of no account, but it can accomplish nearly everything or destroy it!" (James 3:5)

Scriptures are very clear about warning you to be careful what comes from your mouth. Wars have begun, and children have been forever wounded by terrible words that they believed to be true.

The speech center is the dominion center for our lives. Our words will make us or break us. Our words determine our boundaries. Our words can limit us or loose us.

If we keep telling ourselves that we can't lose weight, we

will not lose weight. Begin to tell yourself out loud that you will lose weight and put only healthy things into your mouth.

"By your words you shall be justified and **by your words** you shall be condemned." (Matthew 12:37)

If all you ever say about yourself is negative, it will set you up for failure. Your best friend or worst enemy is what comes from your mouth.

> *"Whoever shall* **say**...*he shall have whatever* **he says**.*"*
> (Mark 11:23)

You may feel strange saying positive words out loud to yourself, but try it diligently for one month. Do it in your car when you are alone, or take a walk where no one will hear you and speak positive words out loud. Words are power. You must not only think positive thoughts, you must repeat them out loud to have a positive effect on your body chemistry. What you say out loud creates reality. Just thinking about it may not bring it to pass. After days of repeating truths that are spoken out loud and hearing yourself say them, you will find that you actually begin believing yourself. You are then on your way to changing your life. You must voice **out loud** to make your reality change.

Many successful people not only visualize their success beforehand, but they talk about their success as if it has already happened, and create their own future in the process.

You are the master of your own destiny. Remember, this is about having a positive effect on your body chemistry. You are worth it!

Practice saying the following out loud:

- I will achieve my weight loss goals and maintain my weight at ___ (fill in the blank).

- I love nutritious foods and eating healthy.

- I will not put poisonous substances into my mouth (cigarettes, harmful drugs, processed sugar, artificial sugar, and so on).

- My health is very important to me.

- Junk food has no power over me because I crave fresh fruit, vegetables, lean meat, and whole-grain products.

- I eat green and yellow vegetables and fresh fruit because it keeps my body functioning at its peak.

- I love to exercise because it increases my strength and endurance and pushes back the onset of "old age."

- I find the time to exercise many times per week doing strength training and heart-strengthening exercises because it helps me function better, while increasing my metabolism and improving my health.

- I will not allow anyone, including myself and my well-meaning family, spouse, or friends, to deter me from a healthy lifestyle.

- I will plan ahead and keep healthy foods on hand, at work, and in my home.

- I love drinking water because my body needs plenty for maximum health.

You cannot prove something does not work unless you are willing to put it to a fair test. I double dare you to use this on yourself daily and say "out loud" positive things for one month. See if they don't shape your vision of your future.

Make a list of all the positive things you need to change in your life, and begin saying them out loud several times per day. What comes out of your mouth, you start to believe, and what you truly believe, you will begin to do!

CHAPTER 8

Alcohol Is Not for the Obese

"Addictions are begun in ignorance and end when
we seek something better."

I F YOU ARE WATCHING your carbohydrate intake, alcohol consumption is not helping. You may never lose weight if you continue to enjoy more than an occasional small drink.

Alcohol is quite high in calories, especially compared to carbohydrates and protein:

Carbohydrates or Protein	= 4 calories per gram
Alcohol	= 7 calories per gram
Fat	= 9 calories per gram

Alcohol is absorbed into your bloodstream almost immediately, so **it does not have a filling effect on you and it *slows down your metabolism for as long as three days*. If you are serious about losing weight, skip the alcohol.**

CHAPTER 9

Smokers, We Love You, *Butt*!

"If you start it, you can finish it."

I F YOU ARE A smoker, you have a difficult habit to break. Concentrate on breaking one bad habit at a time so you don't become overwhelmed. You can do it!

When California passed a law to prevent smoking in the workplace, I breathed a huge sigh of relief. My lungs hurt each day after breathing secondhand smoke at the office. Even though I didn't smoke, the smokers were forcing me to breathe their poison and I resented it. My clothes and hair stunk from their self-made addiction, and every evening I couldn't wait to get home and take a shower to wash it out of my hair and get the smell off my clothes.

Unfortunately, I had no way to wash the cigarette smoke out of my lungs. Smokers were forcing their poor choices on me. If you are a smoker, please show respect for others. Don't bother asking nonsmokers if you can smoke in front of them. By doing so, you are letting them know that they are not important to you, and you really don't care about injuring their health, even if they give you permission to smoke. They are being passive at the expense of their own health because they care about you or are afraid of losing their job or because they don't want to be offensive to you. Why not show them how much you care by smoking elsewhere and not being offensive?

Your Smoking Days

Lung cancer from smoking or the effects of secondhand smoke is the leading cause of cancer death in women.

Ex-smokers can be reassured that after passing a decade puff-free, their risk of lung cancer is about the same as that of someone who never smoked. Unfortunately, lung damage from emphysema or bronchitis can't be reversed, but your cardiovascular system can bounce back. The longer you go without smoking, the less will be your risk of heart disease and some cancers.

Although everyone should eat many servings of fruits and vegetables a day, ex-smokers should consider making one or two of those servings strawberries or black or red raspberries, which may prevent the onset of esophageal cancer. Folate (found in whole grains and greens) and B12 (in meat and dairy products) can reduce cell damage that may lead to cancer.

Despite all the hoopla about "safer" cigarettes—low-tar and low-nicotine cigarettes that are supposed to contain fewer toxic substances—they don't exist. For many years, people have taken comfort in the fact that they're smoking low-tar or low-nicotine brands. However, these "healthier" cigarettes demonstrate that low-tar and low-nicotine smokers smoke more cigarettes and inhale more deeply to compensate for the reduced nicotine per cigarette.

A major part of the tobacco addiction game is maintaining a steady level of nicotine in the blood. This is why you think about and reach for a cigarette first thing in the morning. The longer the time between cigarettes, the lower your blood nicotine level dips. You feel this as increasing nicotine-withdrawal symptoms. If you smoke a low-nicotine brand, you will either inhale more deeply or smoke more often to equal the amount of nicotine you would be getting from regular cigarettes.

Regardless of the type of tobacco you use, the stuff kills you prematurely.

Repeated doses of nicotine cause a general overload of the nervous and cardiovascular systems. Blood vessels clamp down in response to this repeated chemical assault. Narrower, constricted blood vessels lead to elevated blood pressure and a greater likelihood of obstructions to circulation.

In the human body, dangerous backups, bleeds, hemorrhages, and infarcts occur. Infarcts are cell deaths resulting from the cutting off of the blood/oxygen supply. Long-term construction of blood vessels and increased blood pressure also lead to increased formation of atheromas, which are fatty deposits that form right beneath the delicate inner lining of blood vessels. Atheromas clog the pipe, which may end up as a life-threatening blockage in an artery of the heart or brain.

Although your body is fully capable of recognizing and fighting off thousands of microorganisms and toxins, your immune system can become overwhelmed. **One sign of immune system burnout is frequent or persistent infections, such as upper respiratory infections and colds.**

When you use tobacco, you end up swallowing some of the smoke and/or tobacco and associated particulate matter. Like the lining of your mouth and intestines, the gastric mucosa can react to repeated contact with tobacco carcinogens by forming mutated (cancerous) cells and breaking down the gastric lining. This results in peptic ulcer disease.

The constituents for tobacco smoke that make it from your lungs into your bloodstream pass through your kidneys, which filter the blood and excrete these toxins into the urine. Urine that contains carcinogens sits in the bladder for hours at a time—a setup for bladder cancer.

Your liver, which is the recycling plant of your body, ordinarily breaks down thousands of chemical compounds, including tobacco compounds that pass through your gut and bloodstream every day.

Men and women who smoke lower their chances of successfully conceiving a child because fertility decreases.

Smoking boosts the risk of lung, bladder, pancreatic, cervical, and other cancers, as well as emphysema and chronic obstructive pulmonary disease. It's been linked to infertility, miscarriage, asthma, stroke, low birth weight deliveries, and more severe menopause symptoms. Smoking just one cigarette has been known to trigger heart attacks. Reading the warning label on a pack of cigarettes should scare you into quitting. Smoking ages individuals at an astonishing rate; deep wrinkles appear at a much younger age.

Quitting smoking is the number one benefit you can do to improve your health immediately.

Today there are smoking cessation tools on the market. Wanting to badly enough is the key. You will have to will yourself through those first few weeks of the addiction withdrawals until you find freedom at last from this death grip on your life. You and your family are worth it.

As a smoker, you may spend $10 or more per day ($3,650 per year) on a habit you often hate and that pollutes the air and gradually suffocates you or even kills you before your time. Your health insurance costs keep climbing, partly because of the billions of dollars needed to diagnose and treat lung disease and other medical complications of tobacco use. You are literally burning your life and dollars into smoke.

A Michigan couple recently received a $4,000 bill in past due tax charges from the IRS because they ordered their cigarettes on-line and did not pay their state sales tax. They were given only thirty days to pay up. Ouch!

Diabetes of any kind, heart disease, and strokes occur much more frequently in the smoker because your body is working overtime trying to rid itself of the hundreds of poisonous chemical toxins.

My dad smoked for forty years. We could hear him coughing his lungs out night after night and year after year, coughing so hard that his back would spasm and he would lie in traction or under a heat lamp for days. One night he coughed up blood and made the choice to quit smoking immediately. He never smoked again, but he coughed up stuff for the next forty years of his life suffering from emphysema. It was embarrassing and nauseous to be around him because it made some of us in his presence reflexively gag. Every visit to him in his old age led to our having to suppress vomiting reflexes while trying to balance mind over matter after witnessing thousands of his lung-disgorging episodes.

I'm not telling my family history to disgust you but to put it upon your heart that this is not a pleasant way for family members to remember you. This is not a healthy legacy to pass to your children, but they will become addicted to smoke if you smoke in the home, in the car with them, or anywhere else that they are a prisoner in your jail of addiction. Therefore, you have made them a nicotine addict without their input.

CHAPTER 10

Muscle Building and Heart-Strengthening Exercise

"It's easier to give up, but that's a poor habit."

I F YOU DON'T COMMIT to serious, consistent exercise, then you cannot expect to lose much weight or keep it off. Dedicate at least three episodes weekly, twenty minutes each, of hard aerobic exercise routines (swimming, dancing, jogging, hiking, fast-paced walking, marching), or your metabolism will remain sluggish. In addition to that, set aside at least twenty minutes twice a week for weight-resistance training to build your muscle mass and keep it. Some machines allow you to do both anaerobic and aerobic exercises at the same time (for example, stair stepper machines or simply climbing up and down steps will both strengthen leg muscles and help your cardiovascular system). You also need to build and tone the upper body muscles and lower back muscles with some form of exercise. More often is more effective, but build slowly if you are out of shape and have not exercised in years. The more effort you put forth, the more active and revved up your fat-burning abilities will become.

Give yourself permission to take one day off per week from planned exercise to keep balance in your life. Some people spend hours each day at the gym, working out judiciously or jogging an hour every day. Your body needs time for healing. Overexercising can actually lead to muscle strain and exhaustion. Most of us don't have trouble with too much exercise; our problem is starting.

Why Should I Be Active?

Physical activity can bring you many health benefits. People who participate in moderate-intensity or vigorous-intensity physical activity on a regular basis benefit by lowering their risk of developing coronary heart disease, stroke, type two diabetes, high blood pressure, and colon cancer. Additionally, active people have lower premature death rates than people who are the least active. **A lack of physical activity can hurt your health**.

Regular physical activity improves health and reduces the risk of premature death in the following ways:

- Reduces the risk of developing heart disease, heart attacks, and stroke

- Lowers both total blood cholesterol and triglycerides and increases the "good" cholesterol

- Lowers the risk of developing high blood pressure

- Helps reduce blood pressure in people who already have hypertension

- Lowers the risk of developing non-insulin-dependent (type two) diabetes

- Reduces the risk of developing colon cancer

- Helps people achieve and maintain a healthy body weight

- Reduces feelings of depression, anxiety, and stress

- Helps build and maintain healthy bones, muscles, and joints

- Helps older adults become stronger and better able to move without falling or becoming excessively fatigued

- Helps people with attention deficit hyperactivity disorder focus and concentrate longer.

The Importance of Physical Activity

People of all ages who are generally inactive can improve their health and well-being by becoming active on a regular basis.

Exercise substantially reduces the risk of dying early, offers fewer days spent in the hospital or doctors offices, and reduces the dependency on medications. Moreover, physical activity need not be strenuous to be beneficial; people of all ages benefit from participating in regular, moderate-intensity physical activity, such as twenty to thirty minutes of **brisk** walking five or more times a week. Lollygagging on your walk will do little to raise your metabolism. You've got to move with gusto and enthusiasm while working up a sweat to get your heart rate up.

Despite the proven benefits of physical activity, most of my fellow citizens do not get enough physical activity to provide health benefits. Too many of us sit on our duffs during leisure time instead of getting out there and moving.

Unfortunately, many schools in our new age of supposed enlightenment do not promote physical activities for middle school and high schools. If physical education is not required, then a large percentage of children do not participate, to their own detriment. **As liability rates soar, many schools have cancelled exercise altogether.**

Exercise helps prevent disability as you age. It's also a key factor in overall longevity. People with the highest level of physical activity live longer and spend less time in health institutions.

If you are just beginning an exercise program, start slowly. Don't push yourself so hard that your muscles ache for days. That will only discourage you from further exercise. You are trying to develop a lifetime habit, so make it as enjoyable as possible for yourself. Over the first few weeks, you'll be amazed at how quickly you'll snap into better shape. After that, your progress may be a bit slower. Set realistic goals for yourself, and remember that you're not training for a marathon. Don't lift weights every day, or your muscles will not have time to heal in between sessions. Do at least two or three times per week (but not consecutive days) for lifting weights or any type of resistance training. Resistance training every day leads to sore muscles. You need days between for healing purposes.

When you exercise, expect a normal rise in your pulse rate. If you feel dizzy, have chest pains, or feel very short of breath, *stop*. Check things out with your doctor before you exercise to that level again. You want to know whether your arteries are so clogged that you could keel over from a heart attack or stroke with minimal exercise. People who are in shape and have consistently exercised all of their lives have reduced their possibility of a heart attack even if their arteries are partially clogged, because their arteries have more elasticity. Avoid exercising outdoors in extremely hot or cold weather. When the weather is against you, you can walk at your local mall or put on some fast music and dance, or march indoors.

Lift weights to lower your weight. The more muscle you have, the higher your metabolism rate. In fact, extra muscle increases your metabolism even when you're at rest.

Shoveling Snow

Every winter, people in their thirties and forties keel over dead while shoveling snow. Shoveling (like lifting weights) can raise your heart rate **and blood pressure** dramatically, so pace yourself. I've learned to slow down after hearing those grim statistics. If you don't exercise unless you're forced, then hire the neighbor's kid to shovel snow. Even if you are in good physical shape from a consistent exercise program, shovel a few scoops and pause to enjoy the scenery, wave to the neighbors, or watch the snow fall. This gives your heart time to rest. Without realizing it, you may just shovel away, your heart will speed up, your blood pressure will skyrocket, and the cold weather may possibly have a deadly effect on your overexertion.

Lift Away Pain

Use your back muscles in your exercise program to keep those muscles strong. You will have fewer back injuries and spend less time at the doctor's office when your back muscles are well developed. Concentrate especially on those exercises that strengthen your lower back and abdominal muscles. These are the muscles you lift with and that seem to cause the most problems if weak.

Exercise to Decrease Breast Cancer

Active workouts have been found to protect against and lower the odds of breast cancer.

Old-Fashioned Fitness

Our great-grandparents ate phenomenal amounts of meat and potatoes, smothered with grease-filled gravy, and never went to the gym. Why were they so fit? The answer is in their activity level and their lack of prepackaged junk foods. Their meat was lean from range-fed livestock that weren't locked into tiny cages or shot full of fast-growing hormones. Everything our ancestors ate was used up to produce energy to complement their activities. They walked tremendous distances in a day just to feed the chickens in a building that was a distance from the barn and house. They walked to milk the cows, feed the cows, shovel manure, and tend to their huge garden plots, where they planted, watered, and weeded. They carried bucket after bucket of water out to their gardens and back to the chicken house and livestock barns for the animals. If the wind wasn't blowing to activate the old windmill, they hand-cranked the water up from the well to fill the tank for the cattle and chopped the ice out every winter with a pickax to do it all over again the next day. Several hours per week, they used long, curved knives to "mow" the grass around their homes or more recently a push mower. The children lived in a safer world and walked miles to school and back every day.

Nowadays most people "turtle up" inside their dwellings and never venture outside all weekend unless it's to jump in their cars to shop or eat out. The most activity they get may be walking from the remote control to the bathroom and refrigerator.

Heart Healthy Exercise

If you adopt just one healthy lifestyle change to cut your risk for killer heart attacks and strokes, make sure it's regular physical activity. Exercise can increase "good" HDL cholesterol, zap "bad-guy" LDLs, reduce the risk of fatal blood clots, lower blood pressure, and make muscles more sensitive to insulin—all of which lower the risk of heart attacks.

Men Lose Faster

Yes, men lose weight faster and more easily than women, so get over it! It's muscle that burns fat. Generally, *men have about 30 percent more muscle mass* **than a woman of equal weight and height**. In the race for weight loss, men automatically have unfair advantage.

Build Muscle Mass to Burn Calories

Women, if you want to lose weight, you must build and keep your muscle mass. There are training instructors at almost every gym across the country who will introduce you to muscle-building equipment, or you can purchase your own. Libraries are filled with fitness books you can check out for free and use to build your own exercise routine. There are many decent strength-building machines available. Check out garage sales or your local sports shops for the latest exercise equipment.

Test it on location and see if it's something that will work for you. If you are serious enough to exercise, you may want to purchase your own gear. Stretch bands or a BodyBow used for weight-resistance training are very inexpensive and provide a great way to increase muscle mass. Also they are lightweight and easy to transport. Small barbells are inexpensive, or you can use heavy books or resealable storage bags filled with water.

I plateaued for months at 160 pounds, where I felt good but was still carrying large amounts of excess fat hidden beneath my size fourteen clothes. I chose to just enjoy the journey instead of becoming overly anxious. I continued to eat healthy and increased my muscle-building exercise routines. Even when weight loss slows or maintains, that is far better than the alternative of gaining. Eventually, my weight began to drop again. It's as though my body had to make some chemical adjustments to the lower amount of fat mass. As you lose weight, you won't need as much food to maintain your shrinking mass. Ideally, your appetite will also drop in proportion to your weight loss.

Plan a walking route and push yourself to move faster each week. Find a flight of steps that you can run up and down until you are dripping with sweat. Climbing stairs not only is an excellent aerobic exercise but also builds your leg muscles. Muscle burns fat! Lift heavy books up and down in all directions to build muscles in your arms and shoulders. You can jump rope at home if you have enough space. Pace the floor while you're listening to the television. If you don't live in an area conducive to safe neighborhood walks, take up dancing or marching in place. Put on your favorite fast-paced music and just *move*! Anything is better than sitting hour after hour watching television. Small changes lead to bigger changes. If you have the desire, you can find the way.

Self-Paralysis

The average American watches television over five hours per day. If you are one of those self-induced, paralyzed couch potatoes, this equates to over 1,825 hours per year. If you have watched that much television from the time you were three until you are seventy years old, this equates to fourteen years of sitting on the sidelines watching other people living life. Think of what you could have accomplished by reading, studying, taking classes, or exercising. Think of the pounds you would not have gained, had you stuck to an exercise regime day after day, week after week, year after year. Make a commitment now to spend less time wasting time and more hours furthering your education and fitness level.

If you have not been exercising consistently up to now, could you survive a workout? Your muscles are soft and flabby, and your heart and other muscles might easily become stressed with too much too soon. Get a physical if you have any doubts, and find out what shape you've really gotten yourself into. Ease into the exercise gradually so you don't tear muscles or become overly exhausted. Increase your time and speed weekly until you no longer feel the impact, and increase it each time it begins to feel too easy.

For optimum health, do exercises that increase your heart activity such as running, fast dancing, swimming laps, climbing stairs, or fast-paced walking, as well as exercises that increase your muscle mass. Do these exercises a minimum of twenty minutes nonstop three times per week, but preferably five or six times per week if you want to make progress. Find something you enjoy, and chances are you will stick with it. The more you move, the more you will burn calories. The more often and more consistently and intensely you do your workouts, the faster you will lose weight. After just two or three weeks, you will feel stronger and more energetic. You will sleep better.

We begin to lose muscle mass as early as our twenties **if we are not doing some form of weight-resistance exercise**. As we lose muscle, our metabolism slows down. Every pound of muscle burns thirty-five to forty calories per day, while one pound of fat only burns **two calories**. Think about that: if the average woman has only 10 pounds of muscle in her entire body, she will burn an extra 350 calories per day. This may not seem like much, but over a year's time you have saved yourself from gaining about thirty-five pounds of fat. As we age, it is easy to gain weight and get fatter if we don't exercise. The thin muscles that were holding your waistline in place now turn to fat, which takes up more space than muscle, even if you don't gain any weight. You will want to keep what muscle you already have plus add more.

Many of today's children have little opportunity to develop a healthy amount of muscle in their growing years. They live in inner cities with no yards in which to play and no physical activities in their schools. They are being set up for a lifetime of weight-control failure and ill health. It is the parent's responsibility to get your children involved in physical activities that they will enjoy.

Muscle-building exercises should be aimed at increasing and strengthening the muscles in three main areas of your body: your arms and chest, abs and lower back, and leg muscles.

For your arms and chest muscles, lift small barbells (or heavy books) slowly in all directions over your head, outward from your body and straight up in front and to the side and to the rear. Lift in each direction slowly at least ten times. Begin with small enough weights that you don't tear muscles or ligaments. Coming from an active farm background, I use ten-pound weights in each hand, but this would tear muscles and stress ligaments in arms that are not fit or used to such resistance. Most women are more comfortable with three to five pounds. If you can afford a machine like the Bowflex or use one in a gym, this helps you do all the muscle-resistance exercises you need to strengthen your arms, torso, legs, abs, and lower back.

To tighten your abs and lower back muscles without spending a cent, nothing beats lying on something comfortable as you face the ceiling and doing the following:

- While keeping your head and shoulders straight (don't jerk your neck), lift your head and shoulders slowly off the floor as far as you can and hold for a few seconds. Then lower yourself slowly back to the surface and repeat until you can't do it anymore. Keep your hands at your sides. You will feel your stomach muscles tighten.

- Lie on your back and lift your legs slowly without bending your knees until they are facing the ceiling. Lower very slowly and you will feel your muscles screaming in every direction. Keep this up until you can't do it any more.

These two exercises alone will strengthen those tummy and lower back muscles. Work up to fifty repetitions of these exercises three times per week. If you are excessively heavy or out of shape, you may have trouble finishing one or two. Every day strive to do one more set as you gain strength and make awesome progress. If you need to rest between each set, rest for a few seconds and make yourself do one more. You are not in a race. You are building strength and endurance; it doesn't matter how long it takes.

A great leg muscle-strengthening exercise is stair climbing. It costs nothing and is highly effective. If you can only make it up and down one flight of ten steps, then make it your goal to work on two flights and so on, until you find yourself increasing in strength and endurance. By the end of six months or one year, set a goal of climbing ten steps ten times in a row and back down again. Running up a flight of ten to twenty steps will reveal how well your lungs and heart are working and how much work is ahead of you.

Another exercise for your legs is to stand up and march in place or around the room, lifting your knees as high as you can. If you are extremely overweight, you may not be able to do ten sets. Increase your routines until you can easily do fifty in one session. Lift your knees as high as possible.

To increase flexibility and lower risk of leg injuries, do the following stretching exercises several times per week:

Face a table or back of a chair to hold for support. Lift each leg to the side until it is at least ninety degrees to your body ten times and lower slowly. Lift each leg to the rear until it is ninety degrees to your body at least ten times and lower slowly. Lift each leg to the front of you until it is ninety degrees to your body at least ten times and lower slowly.

My mother was one of the world's most active farm women, but I distinctly remember her doing stretching exercises daily in spite of nonstop chores and farming activities that needed to be accomplished to maintain our way of life. It helped keep her limber and flexible.

When living in ice and snow country, it is very important to keep limber and flexible. Sometimes the frost or ice will cause legs to slip out from under you at very odd angles. Because my muscles are used to being stretched in all directions, there is less risk of injury.

Five Pounds of Muscle Is Skinnier Than Five Pounds of Fat

Yes, it is true. Though both weigh five pounds, muscle is denser and takes up less space in your body than fat. Muscle burns more calories.

Women who consistently do the triple series of exercises to strengthen arms, legs, and torso might gain at most several pounds of muscle, but they will also become leaner and burn more calories in a day. Their bodies will become tighter and more compact instead of flabby. Rarely do women add more than an extra three to five pounds of muscle with consistent workouts unless they are committed bodybuilders who lift huge weights. If you have never done any strength-building exercises, you are in for a surprise. Your waist will tighten, you will notice strength increasing in your arms and legs, and you will feel stronger and more capable. You might experience no weight loss while you are building muscle mass or seem to be losing much more slowly than you hoped, but your jeans will be loose around your waist and inches will disappear from your body mass. Remember, you are building a lifestyle and improving your strength and health. You are not in a race; you are building healthy habits.

Exercising not only burns calories while you are doing it, but it also keeps your metabolism elevated to burn more calories for hours.

The Pomeranian Factor

My Pomeranian burns calories at an incredible rate. Pound for pound, she can outeat our more relaxed, eighty-pound retriever. She is high-strung, burns off nervous energy by challenging all comers, and does her best to terrorize strangers who come near our home. The other day, this tiny ball of fluff escaped past me and chased two teenagers on inline skates down the road. She will fight over her turf, toys, and bones, and never cries "Uncle," even if the larger dog pins her down. Once released, she will rise up on her hind legs, looking all the part of a seasoned boxer, facing the jaws of the larger dog, all the while biting hard with her sharp needlelike teeth and demanding respect. Generally, the larger dog tires of the confrontation and eventually lets our pom have her way. She is relentless and will not give up.

It's the family joke that we got this small dog because she doesn't eat much, when in reality she can match us bite for bite at the dinner table and will take scraps of food from all six of us and still scarf up every table scrap the baby drops or purposefully throws to her. All of this luxury food is in addition to the scientifically well-balanced dog kibble to which she has unlimited access. Even when she's sleeping, she is a terror to behold if we dare shake the covers while entering or exiting her bed. She will leap up from a sound sleep snarling and fighting mad, ready to do battle with the imaginary monster or pounce with fangs on the unknown enemy lurking beneath the blankets. She has never suffered from being overweight. Her metabolism is high, and she burns off her excess calories.

Homegrown Exercise or the Gym

Personally, I don't enjoy the time or effort it takes to drive to a gym, use grimy equipment that thousands of other people have handled, shower in a strange facility, or get back into my car drenched in sweat. For the price of one or two year's worth of club memberships, I own several simple and inexpensive exercise machines. I have the discipline and motivation to use my personal exercise equipment. In earlier years, I walked fast for miles every evening after work and weekends in decent weather. For muscle resistance, I used two barbells that I lifted up and down in all directions with my arms. Though I struggled with weight during those years, I know that consistent exercise kept me from gaining significant poundage. The benefits of extra muscle mass and weight-resistance training was not as well known in those years.

My daughter, on the other hand, prefers the gym membership. It's her way of getting uninterrupted, quality exercise time away from the constant interruptions of ringing phones, kids, knocks on the door, and so on. It's her time to listen to educational tapes undisturbed.

If you can stand on your feet and move your arms and legs, you can exercise. If you are physically challenged but have use of only one or two limbs, exercise those limbs as often as possible to the maximum of your ability. If you're a quadriplegic, exercise your mind and eat proper nutrition to keep it sharp. Do what you are capable of doing, and don't bother with what you can't do.

My granddaughter once asked me why I hike the nine-mile trail, and I told her "Because I can." If you don't use it, you will lose it. Shake it, roll it, stretch it, and move it! My goal was to hike that nine-mile trail around a nearby lake, but I could only dream about it at 200 pounds. While I was dropping from 200 to 175, I walked the neighborhood, building strength and getting in shape. I attempted and accomplished that trail for the first time at 175 pounds. Before that, my legs and back hurt too much. Once on that trail, there was no shortcut back unless I swam the lake. At 175 pounds, I conquered the trail without my legs aching for hours. I took several breaks and babied a few blisters on my feet, but that pretty much wiped me out for the day. I continued those long hikes with heavier socks while losing weight, and it got easier each weekend. How many people my age are slowing down, reducing their activity, and taking it easy clicking a remote while never breaking a sweat?

After recovering from that starvation diet in my teens, I remember needing more naps. Eating seemed to be the only way to feel better, so I gained back forty-four pounds in two years. The only reason I didn't replace that weight quicker was because of my extreme activity level with farm chores. I tossed heavy bales of hay around and shoveled a ton of feed daily from the silo for the cattle, and then scooped it into a bushel basket and made numerous trips to the feeding trough every day. Spare time was spent hiking around our 160-acre farm for fun and swimming at the local pool for hours. I also rode my bicycle for miles around the countryside, including fourteen miles round-trip to our second farm, where I worked during the summer months herding sheep (on my feet all day) along the roadside ditches. There was always that muskrat nest to check out in the creek up the road, ice-skating on the nearby lake, snowdrifts to play in, and snow tunnels to dig. I used to shovel out our entire long rural driveway after each snowfall just for fun as a teenager and mow an acre of land during the summer around all of our farm buildings. Without television or computers, it's amazing what your teenagers will do to keep themselves busy. I shoveled out enough manure from chicken coops and cow stalls to fertilize Rhode Island.

During northern winters in those earlier years, snow came down in feet, not inches; this was before global warming changed our weather patterns significantly. Each day we had livestock to tend and water, ice to break in the livestock tank, grain to haul in buckets, hay to stack, weeds to pull, grain and chopped corn to shovel, and manure to pitch.

Being physically active will keep you from gaining volumes of weight if you are eating poorly, but **when you eat nutritiously and responsibly, the nutrients will help you achieve your weight goals without as much effort**.

Currently, my exercise routine at home includes listening to favorite programs or CDs because it allows me to do two things at once and the time passes quickly. I do both aerobic workouts (hard breathing) and anaerobic weight-resistance workouts (building muscle).

The time of day you choose is key to your success. For myself, I exercise first thing in the morning in my pajamas before showering or eating. This saves me time by not having to shower or change clothes twice. It helps fire up my metabolism first so I will burn more calories all day. Early morning is the time when I am least interrupted by grandchildren, phone calls, work, or family-related obligations. In good weather, I'm out at the crack of dawn hiking and back home soon enough to have the entire day left to accomplish other weekend commitments.

When traveling, I stick to an exercise routine by rising early and pacing the hallway in the hotel for thirty minutes of walking and doing some stretching exercises before breakfast. Weight-resistant stretch bands are lightweight and perfect for travel. They help keep muscles from atrophying for any long periods away from home.

When my sisters and I get together, we enjoy hiking. One sister travels globally in her career and keeps a walking meter to monitor how many steps she takes daily to get in her goal of so many thousands of steps. My oldest sister and her spouse bicycle for miles. They've been in thirty- to sixty-mile marathons in recent years. They set their own pace and plan on enjoying the scenery and points of interest along the route instead of just pressing metal to be the first to finish. They are also in their seventies, and their active lifestyle has kept them young. They proudly speak of the people in their eighties who are active in these bicycle marathons. If you want to be active in your old age, begin now. What you do today will either lay the groundwork for an active or "rocking chair" retirement. You are making the choices for your future body today! An exercise program should include things you enjoy. If you enjoy your workouts, you will look forward to them.

My son-in-law has a grandmother who recently flew from her home in Hawaii to Las Vegas to celebrate her ninetieth birthday with a dear friend. His other very active grandmother is in her late eighties and can be spotted daily in her small town because she is living life, not sitting at home waiting for the end. The grim reaper has stopped by her door several times and was told in no uncertain terms that she wasn't ready! Every choice you make is either helping you live life to the fullest or pulling you one step closer to your grave.

Don't Discourage Yourself with the Wrong Mentors

Exercise instructors with unattainable bodies may leave you discouraged before you begin. Choose mentors whose bodies you can relate to.

One reason Mary Lou Retton (Olympic gymnast) was so popular is because she was not your typical gaunt gymnast. She won her place on our U.S. Olympic team because someone else on her team was injured before the Olympics. Mary Lou was a muscular, curvy dynamo who you couldn't stop watching. She became an overnight sensation and Olympic champion. She had a "neon light" grin as large as her talent, and everything she threw herself into, she did with gusto. It defied the laws of gravity for this bombastic, tiny, muscular, well-rounded girl to do the things she did. People could relate to her because she was shaped like the girl next door, your kid sister, or your best friend. Her parents said they enrolled her in gymnastics because she was a child who was bouncing off the furniture with super energy, and they wanted Mary Lou to channel it into something constructive.

Sea Biscuit was the horse that couldn't be beat. He wasn't big enough and didn't look fast enough to have superstar status, but he beat everything that moved because he had the heart.

Do you want to be the best you can be, or are you going to settle for the past and the present and never change anything?

Walk a Shelter Dog

For those who love dogs and live near a local animal shelter, volunteer to walk or jog the dogs. This may be the only chance the animals have to get out while waiting for a new home. What a great feeling it is to exercise while helping a homeless animal enjoy quality time!

Exercise Hard Enough That You Feel It

When you exercise harder, your cells respond by using oxygen at a faster rate and burning more calories. Only hard exercise that increases your heart rate and causes you to break into a sweat will change your metabolism. You will not lose weight if your intensity is not high enough. The more oxygen your body uses, the more calories you are burning. If you think walking slowly is exercising, you are almost wasting your time unless that is all you have the strength for today. You need to push your feet fast, walk hard, swing your arms, and start breathing harder. If it will help you to wear some headphones with Tina Turner songs, then do so. She was still dancing up a storm well into her sixties and is still going strong at the publication date of this book. Tina did not settle for an "easy chair."

When you are exercising properly, you need to be moving fast enough to feel fatigued, but be able to continue this level of exercise through your session without keeling over. You must breathe deeply while still able to carry on a simple conversation if necessary. This type of exercise will burn fat and rev up your metabolism.

Just Do It

Every cell needs oxygen. Walking, running, cross-country skiing, or swimming (not just standing around in water) pushes oxygen into every cell in your body. Your heart rate needs to be elevated to keep your circulation functioning properly. **Without adequate exercise, cells begin to die from lack of oxygen, and muscles begin to atrophy from lack of use**.

I have a habit of pacing the floor while watching TV or while listening to educational CDs or DVDs. I simply can't sit still long enough to watch a thirty-minute program. My large mutt wants me to constantly toss him a ball or tug rope and will not allow me to sit without barking in my face.

Ten Signs It's Time to Change Your Exercise Routine

1. You skip your workouts to watch TV.

2. You own one exercise outfit, but it hasn't been used in years, and they stopped making it in the 1970s.

3. Your hair looks as good at the end of your workout as it did before you started.

4. The last time you changed your routine was during the Nixon administration.

5. You still exercise to the music of "Fame."

6. Of the thirty-six machines at your gym, you've only used one.

7. You think crunches are the funny noises your knees make.

8. You've broken the snooze alarm button trying to get up for an early workout.

9. You don't know the difference between anaerobic and aerobic.

10. You don't need to shower after you "worked out."

As You Age, You Lose Muscle without a Fitness Program

Before your mid-thirties, you start to lose about a half pound of muscle a year (and it can accelerate as you get older). With every pound of muscle lost, your metabolism falls off by burning fewer calories per day. If you're not gaining weight but your clothes are not fitting, it's a sign that you're replacing that muscle with an equal amount of fat, which takes up more space than muscle—a lousy scenario for more than just your wardrobe. This creeping fat loves to hang out around your middle, increasing your risk of developing type two diabetes, heart disease, and even some types of cancer. The sooner you take action to build and keep muscle mass, the better.

Increase Your Metabolism By Drinking Water

We've all been told that most of us are dehydrated and need to drink more water. **Drinking eight glasses of water a day can burn off almost 35,000 calories a year, which is equivalent to about ten pounds of fat. Cool water works best because part of the increased calories burned occurs as your system warms the water to body temperature.**

Water decreases the blood's thickness and lowers the risk of developing heart attacks and dangerous blood clots. Other liquids seem to increase blood's thickness, because water is drawn out of the bloodstream to help digest them. This is why nothing can take the place of water.

One granddaughter has to be constantly reminded to drink water. Without it she suffers from dizziness. Some folks will experience headaches without enough pure, plain water (other drinks don't count).

Be Careful what You Think

What you think can impact your workout almost as much as what you do. Long-distance runners and athletes will tell you it's the power of their minds over their tired bodies that makes them win or lose. Negative thoughts can hurt performance, reduce benefits, and even keep you from exercising as frequently as you should. Insulting yourself won't keep you motivated to exercise better. To increase your chances for success, praise what you do right, such as keeping your eye on the ball or maintaining your balance, rather than focusing on what you do wrong. Concentrating on what you do correctly reinforces those actions. It also makes the sport more fun, so you're likely to be motivated to try again. Replace self-defeating thoughts with positive ones to keep you going and make exercise easier.

What do athletes do? They have persistence and tenacity. They visualize their success. They stick with the program and never give up. No one remembers a quitter.

CHAPTER 11

Plan Ahead

"No plan, no future."

IT IS SAID THAT it takes twenty-one days to solidify a new habit. Set reasonable goals for what you wish to accomplish. Set an attainable weight goal and exercise program for what you plan to achieve, but no time limit, because you do not know how fast or slowly you will lose. This is not a race. It's a time to build health and concentrate on creating lifelong habits. If you don't already have an exercise program established, then begin with three or four workouts per week for thirty minutes each time. Gradually increase the minutes per day and the days per week. If you can't walk around the block, make that your first goal. Break the block barrier, and then begin to increase your walk farther and faster as you become stronger. Break it up into muscle-building and hard-breathing exercise. Pick workout routines you enjoy. If you have fun with your activities, you will stick with them. If you hate exercise, then do it while watching television or listening to your favorite music. Determine to stay with it for twenty-one days. You will feel better, look better, and be on your way to a lifetime habit where nothing will shake you from doing it.

The same holds true for what you need to resist eating. If you are addicted to sugar, like me, swear off sugar or any food that you crave for at least three weeks. Don't restrict yourself in any way on healthy eating. Just concentrate on breaking your addiction first. When you are hungry, eat plenty of lean protein, which fills you up. Include many daily servings of green and yellow vegetables and no more than two to three servings of breads or raw fruits. Also drink plenty of water. During those first two weeks, I was constantly raiding the refrigerator for something to override my sugar cravings. I knifed my way through two pounds of cheese, ate popcorn by the bagful and hundreds of apple slices. I found that after only fourteen days my sugar cravings ceased. After a month off sugar, I noticed that my appetite dropped. **This had never happened in my life** except when I was too sick to eat. Suddenly, I wasn't hungry as often. I didn't need double portions of anything. I could go an entire five hours without eating or even thinking about food. This newfound freedom from cravings and constant hunger was like winning the lottery! I hit the ultimate jackpot in my dieting dilemma. The destructive cycle of dieting and gaining was broken. As long as sugar remained out of my life, I could have a **normal appetite** and lose weight without driving myself insane.

After decades of struggling with my weight and sugar addiction, this was total liberation for me. At first, I cut only the sugar out to stop the unhealthy things it was doing to my body. After my appetite dropped and I began losing weight without dieting, I knew I was on to something wonderful. I continued to enjoy a healthy, balanced diet of lean protein, raw fruits, cooked vegetables, and whole grains. Much to my shock, the weight continued to drop slowly and naturally. In a year's time, I lost about forty pounds without depriving myself or dieting. Sometimes the weight loss slowed and I wondered if I would lose any more, but I was so elated to not be gaining weight or fighting food cravings that I refused to let the time factor bother me. I was just thrilled that the weight was staying off without endless cravings. Also, I noticed other positive changes in my health and well-being. I focused on my newfound health and freedom from addiction. I can't describe to you how it feels to be free from the cravings and to notice that aches and pains have disappeared. You must experience it for yourself.

No longer was I thinking about my next chocolate fix. I was able to concentrate better on my grandchildren and things to do around the house. I wasn't compelled to jump in my car and make the drive across town through a blizzard or driving rainstorm for my "fix." The addiction vaporized. In its place was incredible peace. It was like suddenly being given a gift of focusing on life instead of food. My source of pleasure was no longer sweets. I found that living in itself was precious, where before, I enjoyed life with a dozen chocolate chip cookies or a half gallon of ice cream. I no longer needed to raid the refrigerator for something sweet each time something stressed me, although I still walk by and occasionally open the door looking for something from habit. Habits are hard to break. Since I know I won't be reaching for any sweets (and there are none in my fridge), I close the door and go about my business because I'm not hungry. These are constant reminders of how much I used sugar products as a tranquilizer and crutch for every situation. Now that my blood sugar is stabilized by a healthier lifestyle, common stresses bounce off easily. I don't need my "fix" anymore. Actually, the sugar fix never solved anything. The stresses were still there, and I still had to deal with them whether or not with chocolate in hand.

Idiot rules for dieters are things like the following:

- Use a smaller plate.
- Only eat at the table sitting down.
- Never eat watching television.
- Spend hours cooking.
- Use a smaller fork.
- Eat with a toothpick instead of a fork or spoon.

- Don't eat between meals.
- Do eat between meals.
- Drink water after each bite.
- Chew slowly, and chew each bite thirty-two times before swallowing.
- Eat only this or only that so many times per day.
- Don't eat this, and don't eat that.
- Allow yourself one serving size of dessert with dinner. (Impossible for a sugar addict!)

While those things may help certain people, the only thing I changed and concentrated on that first month was knocking the sugar out of my life. Getting healthy was my first goal. Losing weight just happened along the way by this one dietary change, as I was already on a consistent exercise program.

I have always been a fast eater. Probably it began in my large family environment where we were all competing for food around a kitchen table filled with choices, and mealtime wasn't exactly a pleasant experience. One friend, after watching me eat, said in amazement, "You can slow down; I won't take it away from you!"

Without sugar driving my hunger addiction, my body tells me that I'm full when I'm really full. If I order too much food, I actually leave some on my plate now. No matter how fast or how slowly I eat, my body works properly without the sugar or other unhealthful snack foods. It lets me know when I've had enough.

Mindless eating is keeping you fat. Think before you put something into your mouth.

At first, I merely set my focus on getting through the first month without sweets, but it made such a huge difference in my attitude and health that I have no desire to ever return to that destructive eating cycle. *I don't need sweets anymore.* Their power over me is broken. Without sweets, and by continuing my lifetime exercise regime, my unhealthy cravings dissolved and my weight became manageable without doing anything else. I no longer had to figure it out. All it took for me was to kill those sugar cravings and weight control became easily manageable.

When you start on this journey, don't bring food in the house that tempts you. Your family and children don't need it either. Set an example. You may be impossible to live with while you're getting the cravings out, but it will be worth it. Show your children instead how to peel an orange or cut up a kiwi. Make a game out of it. Make fruit shakes with your blender using nothing but real fruit and packaged frozen fruit to give it that frozen cold texture, along with plenty of water so that it will blend. Set out bunches of grapes or cherries or slices of cheese for snacks.

If there are no healthy places to eat near your place of work, pack your lunch. Make certain you bring meals that will satisfy you, or you will toss them aside and hit the carbohydrate end of the cafeteria. Do your grocery shopping trips after you have eaten, and purchase meals or foods that will transform your work lunches into something you actually enjoy. Always eat some protein before shopping so you won't be tempted to grab an unhealthy snack. After your sugar cravings are gone, these items will no longer appeal to you, but you have to be careful and not tempt yourself until these habits are firmly instilled in your innermost being (about one month). Keep healthy snacks that aren't addictive in your desk drawer at all times in case you notice hunger between meals. I keep a jar full of mixed nuts and another container of pitted dates in my desk. For me, these foods are not addictive. Assorted nuts or dates have tremendous food value, as they are loaded with essential enzymes and minerals. Since I have no problem limiting my quantity of nuts or dates, it does not pose a high-calorie, weight-gaining experience for me. Three or four dates are filling and satisfy my yearning for something sweet; I can easily make it to the next meal without further snacking.

If you travel, plan ahead. Does the hotel serve healthy food? Does it have an exercise room or a pool that you would actually use? Don't settle for a continental breakfast of sweet rolls and coffee. That is heartburn waiting to happen, and you will be hungry again within an hour. It will destroy your resolve by raising your blood sugar levels and will heighten your cravings. Allow yourself time to indulge in a large, healthy breakfast with an omelet and a small glass of real 100 percent juice. You'll be satisfied until lunchtime. If you must order fast food occasionally because of lack of time, pick something with protein and green or yellow vegetables that aren't deep-fried. Choose water or unsweetened iced tea instead of soda or a milk shake. You'll find that you are satisfied until dinner. You won't be so irritable or tired by late afternoon. Allow no sugar to create havoc in your system or elevate your cravings. You'll be able to concentrate on your job better. Warn only those friends and relatives in advance who will be affected by your new eating plan. Don't let anyone talk you out of it. After all, what can be healthier than eating fruits, vegetables, lean meat, and whole grains? Because you are no longer stuffing yourself with sweets, you will find wholesome foods so filling and fibrous that you will eat much less than you expected. Your actual grocery bill should decrease.

Today, if someone at the large company where I work hands me a slice of birthday cake, I discretely dispose of it out of sight of the giver and go on about my business without drawing attention to my sugar-free habits. In my past life, I would have gobbled down my piece and then looked around for seconds.

Add Years to Your life

My resting heart rate dropped over ten beats per minute after losing the extra weight. Longevity has been proven to result from the benefits of a healthy, active lifestyle rich in fruits and vegetables, regular physical activity, a healthy weight, and no smoking.

Step Counters

Get a pedometer from your local sports shop and set a goal of 10,000 to 15,000 steps per day, which is only about two or three miles. You can walk that far in thirty to forty-five minutes.

Lose Weight by Eating More of the Right Foods

Eating small amounts of healthy fat throughout the day can suppress your appetite. Fat signals your brain that you're full. Healthy fat sources are nuts, seeds, and olives. This is another reason why keeping mixed nuts around is so important unless you are allergic to them.

You really can change the foods at your child's birthday parties. Children don't need pop, cake, and cookies. We are turning our children into sugar junkies. There is not one healthy shred of nutrition in that glop of party food, and most of these kids will be bouncing off the walls for hours from the sugar rush. Instead, serve up small glasses of 100 percent grape juice for the kiddies. Most children love grape juice and won't notice the difference or feel that they are somehow being deprived—especially if you plop a small scoop of vanilla ice cream in it, call it a Purple Cow, and hand them a spoon. Set out tiny squares of cheese, as long as no one in the crowd is allergic to dairy, and small triangular sandwiches filled with tuna salad or lunch meat. Give each child a tiny cup of mixed nuts if he or she has a full set of teeth and isn't allergic to nuts. All these foods together will cost you less than one large birthday cake that no one needs. Once you've passed through this first gauntlet with each child, next year it will be even easier because you found that you could change your routine without the world coming to an end.

Before treating our children to the movies, we feed them at home right before leaving and then carry bottled water with us.

The cost and size of the drinks and candies served at theaters will bankrupt you, and your kids don't need it anyway. The size and quantity of sugar in one bag of theater-sized candies and beverage is enough sugar to sweeten your coffee for an entire year. If you fill up your children with nutritious fruits, vegetables, lean protein, and whole grains before they leave home, they won't have any appetite for the sweeter things when you walk past the theater candy counter. After you do this a few times and your children realize that you will not budge on these issues, you have instilled in them the idea that healthy foods are important and you will not waste your hard-earned cash on junk food. It also is teaching them the value of a dollar and keeping them healthier, and you will still have a pocket full of dollars left over that you did not give to the "sugar goddess." If your kids don't see you spending your monies wisely, how can you expect them to? Your example will speak louder to them than anything that you verbalize.

Do you realize that in most children, their health, behavior, and demeanor can change to the positive from proper nutrition? Think what that could do for your outlook!

CHAPTER 12

Laughter and Positive Thinking

"Laughter gives you life."

LAUGHTER REDUCES LEVELS OF certain stress hormones and actually increases our ability to fight disease. Laughing can be a total body workout! Blood pressure is lowered, and there is an increase in vascular blood flow and in oxygenation of the blood, which further assists healing. Laughter also gives your diaphragm and abdominal, respiratory, facial, leg, and back muscles a workout. That's why you often feel exhausted after a long bout of laughing—you've just had an aerobic workout! Laughter also allows you to release harmful emotions such as anger, sadness, and fear, rather than suppressing them.

My mother was always a very serious type, and I made it my mission as a teenager to get her to laugh occasionally. I was born with "happy genes," and life has always been a blast for me. I remember once we were both struggling to carry a heavy seed bag up some steps, and I got her laughing until tears began to roll down her cheeks. It was a rare moment in time that is priceless in my memory.

Who has not heard of the wonderful advances in "laughter medicine" and positive reinforcement games of visualization in children's cancer wards? These tools have produced marvelous effects on the healing of life-threatening diseases. Children and adults have laughed their way out of disease and depression and into health using the power of positive thinking and imagining that the cancer cells (the invaders) are being attacked and defeated by healthy white blood cells (soldiers).

Your mind is the most powerful weapon you have, either to defeat you or to help you achieve each goal you set your mind to accomplish.

Learn to enjoy your experiences today, and try not to take life too seriously. Live for today and what you can accomplish today, and forget worrying about something that may or may not happen tomorrow. Set attainable goals. If you have been a couch potato for years and haven't exercised beyond opening the refrigerator door and clicking a remote, then begin slowly. You may even need to check with your doctor and find out what kind of shape you are really in. Don't get hung up on a scale number. Instead, go by your level of energy and your blood sugars stabilizing, the cravings diminishing, and your clothes becoming loose. This is a lifetime trip, so enjoy the scenery. You didn't become obese overnight. It took years to get yourself in this predicament. Time will continue to pass whether you decide to do anything different or not, so why not begin today at a level that doesn't kill you?

Start by walking around the block. When you can do that without collapsing, increase the distance. When that becomes too easy, power walk and go farther and push yourself harder, but don't overdo it. Slowly build up your endurance and strength so that it will be an enjoyable progression for you, not something you dread.

Breaking through the negative barriers of your mind takes practice until it becomes a habit like anything else. Take the first steps toward your future. Go further than you thought possible. If you are willing to set a new standard for yourself, it will pave the way for other areas of your life. People will enjoy being around you if you enjoy yourself. If you fail to break those mental strongholds of your past, you will continue to travel in circles. It's time to move on and let go of your past hurts and failures. Don't let what happened yesterday determine what you are today. Your feelings of low self-esteem, inferiority, and inadequacy are all in your mind, and your mind can change. Today is the only day you have for sure. You can't change the past, and you don't know what your future holds, but today live at your full potential.

During childhood I had surgery on one of my legs. For many days after the surgery, I hopped around on one foot and used a wheelchair that I remember tipping over several times while leaning too far forward, because I was afraid to put any pressure on my injured leg. My oldest sister gave me a robe and a pair of beautiful blue slippers while I was in the hospital. In my haste to see how wonderful I looked in this new outfit, I stood up and walked over to the mirror. Forgotten was any fear of the pain.

For weeks after that surgery, I limped around and my mother became quite concerned. She asked the doctor at my checkup whether this would be a permanent result of the injury. The doctor chuckled and said, "She can walk without a limp anytime she wants to." After that revelation, I began putting normal weight on both legs. The first time or two I probably winced because I was expecting pain, but then the fear and pain evaporated and I was able to walk normally again. It was simply putting mind over matter. If you believe there will be pain or failure, you may avoid doing what is necessary and you will lose your victory.

Are You Scale-Obsessed?

Do you weigh yourself more than once a day? Do the numbers depress you? Is it the time of the month when your body is holding on to fluids? Did you eat a bag of salted popcorn or three slices of salty pizza the previous evening? If you obsess over the scales, maybe it's time to back off and use other ways to measure how you are doing. Are your clothes becoming loose? Do you feel more muscle tone in your arms and legs?

I weigh every day at dawn and used to stress over fluctuations of 5 pounds when there was no reason for it. It finally dawned on me that my lowest point of the month seemed to only occur once or twice each month. Fluctuations of 5 pounds are normal because so much depends on how much salt you've consumed in various foods. Salt helps retain water or how much waste is being stored temporarily in your intestines. If you are carefully selecting healthy and nutritious foods, there is no reason to obsess because your scale seems to indicate that you gained 4 or 5 pounds since yesterday when you obviously didn't overeat. Now I weigh myself based on that information and don't stress over the 5 or so pounds of fluctuation during the month. I only note the low points of weight on my calendar month to month. If my clothes still fit comfortably, I did not gain fat poundage, only water or waste poundage.

Life is how you wish to view it. Remember how a baby learns to walk. The baby will fall over and over but eventually learns to master the art of walking. Use everything you learn today to build your tomorrows, and you will suddenly find you are the strong one swimming upstream against the current, until you make it to those quiet pools in the shallows.

The Beavers

Did you know that the largest beaver dam on record was over 2,000 feet long? That's about four city blocks in distance. The beavers, who only weigh twenty to forty pounds, built it one stick at a time. Small changes everyday can eventually dam up the mightiest river.

The Toboggan Ride

When I was a teenager, two of my brothers and I went tobogganing with another family of teens on a nearby slope. We went expecting to sled leisurely down this long grade of a hill and out across the field at the bottom until the sled would gradually slide to a stop. All six of us piled on that long toboggan. With a mighty shove from six pairs of hands we flew off the top of that hill, down the slope gathering speed by the second and what we thought would be a quick trip across the field. Soft snow had piled up at the bottom of the hill from a recent storm. When we hit that soft snow with the weight of the sled, we were instantly and completely buried in it, which brought us to a rather sudden, but absolutely soft and quiet stop. The shock of the unexpected end to our slide took us so completely by surprise that we all sat there buried in the snow, unable to move for several seconds, before I started to giggle. Before long, all six of us were laughing uncontrollably at our predicament, and we could do nothing else except laugh ourselves silly for many long minutes. Finally, the guy at the rear was able to back himself up out of the hole and each one of us in turn had to back out as well from the hole until we could pull the empty sled out backwards through the hole in the snow.

My point to this story is that the unexpected on this winter day was so much more fun and exciting than what we had anticipated. It seems that so many things in life fall far short of our hopes and expectations; this time, however, it resulted in a wonderful memory that even now causes me to smile whenever I think of it! By giving up sugar for several weeks, I'm hoping that you too will find much more than you expected in your ability to have easier control in losing weight and what you eat. It's exciting when you notice an unexpected appetite drop to the point that a portion of food lies untouched on your plate. As the months go by, you will try to order the same quantity of food and only be able to finish half of it. Begin today!

All My Problems Will Disappear when I'm Thin

We mistakenly believe that altering our bodies will fix everything. If we fixate on body size as the source of all happiness, and therefore the healer of all wounds, we will be disappointed.

A very common mistake is belief that being thin or at a "perfect number" equals being loved or cherished or being happy. We couldn't be more mistaken. We still need to find a way to live comfortably inside our bodies and make friends with and love ourselves.

You dream about what it will be like when you reach the long-awaited goal. You fantasize about being thin, and you work hard to get there. You are certain that when you arrive, the struggle will have been worth it. Then, at last, you find yourself there—but your new size is just another place, and that's all. Being thin is only the halfway point. You have to keep exercising, eating right, and dealing with the daily stresses of people who already affect you negatively. This lack of finality with food and body size is an ongoing process, not an end point. This is the point where you either shove all your good habits aside and return to a destructive lifestyle of eating whatever you see, or you resolve to continue moving in better choices.

If you are looking for the illusive quality of happiness, this is a separate issue from body size. Attaining your natural weight is an admirable goal, but if your main goal is to be cherished or finding happiness, losing weight won't make it so. Expecting others to bring you happiness is a false hope. You must learn to love yourself. If you think that losing weight will make others love you more, nothing could be further from the truth. They either care for you now, or they don't. You either accept and love yourself now, or you don't. Start to live as though you love yourself. Make a commitment to be kind to yourself every day, and don't badmouth yourself. If you have suffered through any kind of abuse that still affects you mentally today, and you can't seem to shake off the negative aspects of either the abuse or the inability to forgive, I would highly recommend that you read Joyce Meyer's books *Beauty for Ashes* and *Battlefield of the Mind*.

I'm throwing in advice to those of you who haven't found peace or contentment in your life. First key: you must learn to be thankful for all things (when you are being thankful, it's impossible to be negative). Every day write down ten things you are thankful for until it becomes a habit for you to be thankful. When my feet hit the floor in the morning, the first thing that comes into my mind is thankfulness. I'm thankful for the roof over my head and for my pillow and bed. I literally stop and thank God for several minutes for all my blessings before I do anything else. I thank Him for fingers that work, that I'm able to walk and talk, and that I have food in my fridge, a car that gets me to work and back, my job, my kids, and everything else I can think of. Take time every day to thank God and those people who are closest to you, whether it's your spouse, co-worker, or child. Give them honest appreciation for something they have done right. It will keep you from focusing on what they did wrong. Another important key to peace and contentment is to help others by getting involved and donating your time, talent, and finances to worthy and responsible causes. People who are not thankful for their daily bread, shelter, job, or clothes on their back, will never be content with anything else in life, including the size of their body. Losing 300 pounds will not bring you satisfaction if you are not appreciative of your other blessings. If your entire life is out of whack and you just can't seem to get any of the pieces together, it may be time for you to read Joel Osteen's book *Your Best Life Now*. When you are thankful, complaining stops and your entire outlook on life will change.

Be an Optimist

Unfortunately, how you wander through the world—either as an optimist or a pessimist—affects your health significantly.

The worse you feel about yourself and the darker your outlook on life, the worse your health may be and the less likely it is that people will want to be around you. Your outlook and gloom affects others. Your contentment and peace also affect others; they will want to soak in your sunshine.

Be Willing to Pay the Price

You must pay a price to make your goal a reality. Everyone wants to be a winner, but very few people will make the effort to get there.

CHAPTER 13

Slim and Sixty in Sight

"Celebrating without food was a new concept."

AS THE POUNDS MELTED off, I felt the years of heaviness and obesity fall away. Since my cravings were gone, I could now adjust my eating patterns to lose so much easier or simply eat as much as I wanted of healthy foods and not gain. Instead of feeling old, I became twenty in my vitality and energy levels. It's impossible to describe just knowing that I had found the solution to my obesity problem after decades of struggles and actually achieved my weight loss goal. It was so much easier to control what went into my mouth without constant sugar cravings.

The temptation to snack on other useless foods is also something that I must be vigilant about if I want to retain my ideal weight. This means I don't keep potato chips, pretzels, crackers, or other nonhealthy snack foods in my home either.

Your desire to be free of the sugar addiction and to become healthy must be stronger than your desire to remain in your current predicament. You must be willing to fight through the one to two weeks of withdrawals, just as a drug addict must quit the drugs totally to become well. This is the only way to break the power of addiction. Allow yourself at least two months to develop the steady habit of better eating before giving yourself permission to attend the party of the century or eating out at your favorite restaurant that serves the most sumptuous desserts in the universe. You will not be eating those desserts anymore, but that's okay. You won't even crave them. Addicts aren't cured by allowing themselves even one grain of heroin or alcohol, or the addiction continues to keep a stranglehold on its victim. If you continue to allow yourself sugar in your coffee or a scoop of ice cream after dinner, you will never find freedom from this addiction of sweet cravings, and your ability to lose weight or maintain will continue to be extremely difficult, if not impossible. Your future and health will continue to look dismal, indeed.

When people insist that I accept their desserts, I simply state I am too full to eat another bite. I've heard others claim that they were "allergic" to desserts because they knew they would break out in fat!

You really can have a wonderful life after cigarettes, sugar, sweets, salty chips, or whatever your addiction. When I removed sweets totally from my life, I was doing it because it was easier for me to refuse all sweets, than try to control how many bites of sugar calories I could consume each day. Once I had the first taste of a dessert, my cravings took over and it became almost impossible to control. It was to my own surprise and astonishment that sugar cravings can actually disappear in a few days or weeks. In my case, it took two weeks. Evidently, I had never been off sugar long enough in my life for those cravings to subside completely. Without the sugar cravings and the addiction it forms, it gets incredibly easier to control what is going into your mouth. You'll want to eat healthier foods.

Eat the amount of food that makes you feel comfortable. Satisfy your hunger with a variety of delicious choices that appeal to you. You'll find that by cutting out simple carbohydrates from your diet (sugars, desserts, light breads) and substituting lean proteins, fats, and complex carbohydrates (such as fruits, nuts, and vegetables), your appetite will be quickly

172 Martha L. Pekarek

satisfied without thinking about calories, much less counting them. **Overeating is too easy if you eat snack foods (potato chips, crackers, light bread, and sweets).** Eating at least three full meals a day is essential for keeping your blood sugar steady. Include a protein or healthy fruit snack between meals if you find yourself hungry. Over time you will begin to notice that you may even want to skip those in-between meal snacks, depending upon your activity level, because you simply will not be hungry as your appetite drops.

After a year of behaving myself, and when I felt in control of my eating, I found I could even skip an occasional lunch or dinner and barely notice. Sometimes I would be so busy at my job that I would grab only five or six nuts from my desk drawer for lunch and forget all about food until dinner. Sometimes I eat a large lunch and am able to skip dinner entirely because my appetite has changed.

My final seventy pounds of fat loss took about three years to achieve, but it was almost effortless. It has remained off since I stopped eating the substances that were causing the weight gain. I don't have to struggle against the sugar cravings anymore. I don't starve or deprive myself. When hungry, I eat until satisfied. During those three years, I built healthier lifetime eating habits. I do believe that if I could have maintained a harder exercise program, that weight would have come off much faster, but my life revolves around loving three dogs, three grandchildren, a large home and yard to maintain, and a full time job; almost everyone has as many or similar challenges.

Sugar was the nine-hundred-pound monster that controlled my eating behavior in the past. Every gram of sugar would cause unmanageable cravings for more food and would produce constant hunger. This is why it is so important to read labels. If you are a peanut butter maniac, check the sugar content. You may want to switch to old-fashioned peanut butter and add some honey. Some old-fashioned brands come pre-mixed with honey and salt only. For the first year, I avoided honey and molasses because I was not certain how my body would react to their sweetness. Now I use either a spoonful of honey or blackstrap molasses (no processed sugar added) to my hot cereal every morning. Molasses and honey are extremely healthy with vital nutrients, and they do not trigger my overeating responses.

If you are eating five hundred calories of peanut butter or honey every day, then you may need to cease eating these foods.

Ask yourself how many times in the past decade have you lost all the weight you ever wanted to lose and never gained it back. Take a chance for two weeks, and see how much better you think and feel after your sugar addiction cycle is broken and the poison is removed from your system.

You may think that three years is too long to spend losing seventy pounds, but you've probably been trying to lose weight for longer than that while fighting against overwhelming and uncontrollable cravings. Looking for a quick fix is not going to solve a lifestyle of bad eating habits. If you lose your excess pounds quickly and not develop good eating habits along your journey, then you are setting yourself up for failure and a quick regain. All you need to achieve at this point is to get past those first critical weeks of sugar addiction cravings and then be cautious for a few months to avoid temptation until this new habit is fully ingrained. Once those cravings are gone, your weight control will be manageable for the first time in your life. Now that I have learned which foods trigger my cravings (all processed sweets), I merely avoid those and go on about my life. I don't count calories, carbohydrates, or grams. I get three balanced meals per day plus a healthy snack in between when hungry. By not allowing myself to become too hungry, I keep my metabolism high because it takes energy to burn off food calories. That never made sense to me when I was eating too many sugar calories, because at that time I was overwhelming my metabolism with unusable fuel; it had nowhere to put the excess food except into my fat storage cells. Now that I'm eating only healthy foods, my body is able to metabolize and energize properly.

At two hundred pounds I envisioned seven barbells of ten pounds each. As each ten pounds disappeared, I pictured fewer barbells of weight to lose. Several times per week while exercising, I would lift my two ten-pound barbells to remind myself of how much extra weight still remained and how heavy an extra ten pounds is to lift.

Without sweets, the importance of food diminished to a normal means to exist instead of existing to eat. For me, it never worked to try to cut down the amount of sweets. Any amount of concentrated sweets in my body chemistry would trigger the vicious cycle of cravings and hunger. In my former life, I could tell you where every ice cream or frozen yogurt shop was within a twenty-mile radius of my home. I knew where all the Mrs. Field's cookie counters were. Today, not only do I not care, but I'm burning much less gasoline and spending fewer dollars in the process.

If you have a food addiction, go "cold turkey" off sugar (or whatever your addiction is) and the grip will be broken in a very small amount of time—possibly a few days or at most, a few weeks. On one incredible day, it dawned on me that I hadn't thought about chocolate ice cream or cookies in hours. What's more, I hadn't craved them. I was no longer a slave to my sugar addiction. It was an awesome feeling of freedom and power of finally being in control of my appetite. Now I could understand how "normal" people could eat just one cookie and stop. It made me realize that sugar switches an "on button" in my hunger system and doesn't shut off unless I leave it entirely alone. Suddenly, there was no more guilt because I was not eating things that made me feel ashamed, and I wasn't consumed in my thinking about them either. I no longer lived for the next pint-sized milk chocolate ice cream fix or the next plate-sized, melt-in-your-mouth chocolate chip cookie. At last,

I could survive five hours between meals and not even think about food. Hallelujah!

I enjoy life more now because food cravings aren't constantly permeating my brain and interfering with the satisfaction of other areas of my life. There is no further urge to suddenly leave home in the evening to get my favorite pint of creamy milk chocolate to-die-for-ice cream before bedtime. I would actually get irritable if I couldn't get my fix quickly enough. The focus of my weekends stopped being the chocolate sundae at the local mall or the trip past the nearest gourmet cookie counter. Greater pleasure was found in mundane things like taking the car to the repair shop along with a good book. My reading education increased substantially. I read while waiting for that king-sized comforter to wash and dry in the nearby laundromat, instead of raiding the candy machine inside.

More money was left over at the end of the month. My estimate of expenditures for sweetened goodies amounted to at least sixty dollars per month. Some addicts admit to spending several hundred dollars per month on their addictions of sweets or cigarettes. The monetary cost is phenomenal, but the toll on your health is deadly. Another high cost of obesity is your prescription drugs and heartburn medication for alleviating those self-caused problems. These expenses will be greatly reduced, if not obsolete by the end of your weight loss. Being obese is expensive in health and finances. Just getting off one prescription drug may save you hundreds of dollars per year and provide less reliance or need for constant medical attention.

You can only begin to comprehend how **one bad habit negatively affects other areas of your life without even realizing it**, wherein one positive change seeds the way for better things like health, fewer doctor visits, and rare cases of heartburn.

I stopped consuming processed sugar in my diet immediately and totally. If sugar, in any of its various disguises, is listed in the top five ingredients on any package, I refuse to eat it.

I also gave up snack foods that are large on producing weight gain and little on nutrition, such as pretzels, potato chips, and crackers. These items will also cause you to overeat while your body continues to starve for nutrients.

My former eating pattern often consisted of getting half of my daily calories from unhealthy sweets. One large chocolate shake gave me closer to three-fourths of my needed daily supply of calories. Two large slices of pie or cake could easily account for half of my day's calories, but I certainly didn't stop there. After a month off processed sugars, my body was undergoing radical changes, such as feeling better, having less aches and pains, and being in control of my appetite for the first time in my life. From that experience it was easy to determine that this was my new lifestyle and that I was never going back to nonstop cravings. This eliminated self-inflicted aches and pains because of poor eating choices. **It ceased being a temptation because the addiction cycle was broken.**

Much to my surprise, my appetite unexpectedly dropped off. When I began leaving food on my plate, this was a significant milestone in my life. Sometimes I still pile food on my plate from habit but am unable to finish it. Even a greater shock came when month after month, I ate as much as I wanted of healthy foods each day and lost weight at a slow rate of two or three pounds per month. I have never lost weight before without severely decreasing my food intake. Every pound lost felt like a long, drawn out battle that I wasn't meant to win. I could lose a pound and gain three back the next day. What was different this time? The difference was that I was not loading up on processed sugars that immediately became fat storage, and I was less hungry. It was excess sugar that made me excessively hungry all day, even within one hour of consuming a huge meal.

I did not restrict my eating for the first six months, but I continued to eat healthy foods three meals a day and a slice of cheese or one whole fruit or a small handful of nuts in between meals if I noticed hunger. My weight slowly dropped. After that time, I made slight adjustments to eating more lean proteins and vegetables if the weight loss slowed. I never deprived myself or allowed myself to become too hungry.

My health began improving dramatically from the first week. I had fewer colds and coughs, and they were much less severe. After dropping to 175 pounds, my knees stopped hurting and no longer ached at night if I was on my feet all day. I was becoming healthier. My irritability from blood sugar fluctuations disappeared.

At the end of six months, I hit a plateau where my weight loss stalled for two months. I was merely maintaining at this point, which was still a nice change from constant weight fluctuations in the past. I took stock of how much exercise I was actually doing and where I could change my patterns to continue weight loss. Several months earlier, we had brought home a retriever puppy that consumed a large part of my time. The puppy demanded constant attention and in order to keep him quiet so he wouldn't wake up the entire household early in the morning, I played tug of war, toss the ball, and other dog games to the detriment of my exercise program. If I tried to exercise for any length of time, the puppy barked and cried for attention.

After a few months, life settled down into a more fixed routine as the puppy grew into an adult-sized mutt and could entertain himself while I exercised. I cut back on my servings of pastas and breads and instead ate larger portions of lower glycemic vegetables and lean meats. I still ate until I was satisfied and never allowed myself to become too hungry. I stopped eating the raisin bran that had 20 percent sugar content and switched to a health-food store variety of flakes that had no added sugars or sweeteners. I also switched over to eating hot cereal with a teaspoon of blackstrap molasses for sweetener. After making these slight adjustments, my weight continued to decrease. All the while, I was not fighting against cravings.

This was the first time that I found making dietary changes relatively easy. When I was hungry, I ate.

Don't ignore eating when hungry, or your metabolism will decrease in response to what it thinks must be a famine. **In order to conserve energy to survive the "famine," your metabolism will slow to a crawl.**

I was so elated when a size fourteen fit at around 160 pounds. I could feel my collarbone. Plus sizes no longer fit, and my mental health improved when I could shop for average sizes. The large-size catalogs that came in my mail were now trashed without a glance. Boxy outfits that had no shape or style went into the garbage as I shrank in size. There was no purpose in storing fat clothes for future weight gain.

Since I have a short stature by this country's standards, every loss of ten pounds caused me to drop an entire size and resulted in my need for new work outfits. Clothes were too baggy to fit appropriately. I carefully purchased four or five inexpensive outfits to wear on alternating days until it was time to drop into the next size. Then I would shop for four or five more outfits to wear while I waited for the next ten pounds to drop off. Weight loss and gain can be very expensive in the purchase of proper fitting clothing, so I opted for frugality instead of excess. Undergarments, pajamas, and a winter coat were replaced with every twenty-five pounds of loss. A size twenty coat will not keep the winter winds away from a size fourteen individual. It has to fit snugly to hold in the warmth. Even my shoe size changed from nine wide to eight medium at the halfway point. Shoes began falling off my feet, which gave me a clue that my feet were shrinking. Bunions and sore spots on my feet disappeared as shoes fit properly and my own weight decreased, causing fewer pressure points.

One flight of stairs no longer caused my heart rate to speed up.

I stopped gasping for air, and my throat no longer closed off to prevent breathing.

Heartburn disappeared completely unless I allowed myself fruit at the same meal with a spicy dish. My bottle of antacid now sits unused on the shelf where, before my no-sugar life, I was popping them after every meal.

My sleep apnea has virtually disappeared. I did most of the driving for hundreds of miles while vacationing this summer without experiencing any excessive drowsiness. While obese, I could barely keep my eyes open for two miles.

My hands ceased hurting when opening a jar or turning a gas cap.

My chiropractic visits diminished from twice a month to several times per year to keep my spine aligned after an old sledding injury. I keep up back muscle-strengthening exercises because I can bend easier, and my fat no longer gets in the way of movement.

I no longer bite the inside of my cheeks. In my obese life, it was commonplace to bite myself because my cheeks were fat!

My resting heart rate dropped significantly—over ten beats a minute.

My BMI level dropped from almost 40 percent to 24 percent.

My hair grows faster now because of a healthier eating lifestyle.

I can wear any snow boot length because my calves are no longer excessively fat.

Size nine or ten with a stretchy waistband is loose enough for my activity level. It's such a relief to be able to wear clothes with shape and style and use bold colors without stopping traffic. My outfits no longer look matronly, square, or out-of-date.

The large fat deposits that used to hang from various parts of my anatomy are gone. I can actually look down past my belly, see my feet, and still be able to breathe as I bend to trim toenails or pull on socks.

Cleaning my teeth at the dentist office takes less time now. Without sugar, there is no excess buildup of plaque.

My upper arms are no longer excessively heavy, and I'm comfortable being seen sleeveless.

My thighs no longer rub together as I move, and I can see daylight between them.

My hands swing freely past my hips as I walk, and I don't need to hold them away from myself to keep from banging against myself.

My navel stopped being the bottomless pit filled with strange lint and odors to a normal-sized part of my anatomy.

As I drive, there is plenty of room between my belly and the steering wheel, even though my seat has to be far forward for me to reach the pedals.

It's much easier to roll over and get up off the floor. I can now squat to pick up toys and not fall over. I can even get off the floor without using my hands or arms when my hands are covered with sticky stuff from grandchildren.

My nose has shed its extra fat. Who would have thought that noses actually store fat?

I'm startled now by my reflection, as I see a petite person instead of an embarrassingly heavy woman.

I feel twenty years old instead of just old. Carrying all that excess weight was exhausting.

After reaching the midway point, I stopped feeling embarrassment, shame, guilt, and condemnation for the way I looked. I knew I was on the way to my ideal weight, and it was only going to get better. I enjoyed the journey. I was so thrilled with my new health and old aches and pains disappearing, that I did not get discouraged when my weight loss stalled occasionally. I continued to eat when hungry. I ate as much as I wanted of low-carb vegetables and lean meats, along with at least two servings of fruits, and I limited my consumption of breads or pasta. I always ate until I was satisfied. No more starvation diets or deprivation.

Somewhere along the journey I became lax and drifted into eating potato chips every few days because of all the lunch setups that I was doing on my job. My weight climbed seven pounds and remained there until I got serious about letting go of that unhealthy food item.

Food was no longer needed for every personal milestone for celebration. Just "being" and savoring the moment was celebration enough. I finally could feel my rib cage. It was very satisfying, but instead of rejoicing by eating sweets, I partied mentally by just savoring the fact that I was indeed thinner. I often spoke out loud: "I weigh 130 pounds, I eat healthy foods every day, I exercise hard as many times as possible every week, and I am so thankful that I have come this far." It did wonders for my mental attitude, and I believed myself. I was thrilled to not gain weight during this period, but slowly and steadily descended downward on the scales. Losing weight was never so easy. This is the first time in three consecutive years that I did not gain back the weight. Even though I have always been the shortest member of my large family, now I am also the smallest in weight, right where I should be.

I noticed that people treated me differently as I slimmed down. It's as though fat people are not considered worthy of notice or common courtesies. Or it might be that we feel so badly about ourselves that we would rather people didn't notice us.

I am no longer exhausted all day and have boundless energy, which I put to good use. My kids often ask each other where I disappeared and find that I'm out climbing on the roof to remove fallen branches, raking the lawn, weeding the flower beds, or painting the garage.

I can hike around the local nine-mile trail in two hours and fifteen minutes, without pausing for a break, at a steady four-mile-per-hour pace. That's a stiff walk for a middle-aged gal with short legs.

I've recently been described as that "slim girl," which does wonders for my self-esteem, whereas "fat lady" or "heavyset woman" almost caused near hysteria. One cousin referred to me in my past life as being "as wide as she is high."

My blood sugar levels have stabilized, and I no longer fear going into diabetic shock.

I threw out the never-ending journal of my dieting and weight woes. Once I achieved my goal of weight loss and developed three years of healthier eating habits, I trashed years of weight journaling filled with pain and frustration. Now I don't care what I weighed in 1975 or 1992. The only thing that matters now is maintaining the healthy weight that I have and moving toward my future. The months keep rolling by and I still find it easy to maintain.

The only "downside" to my weight loss was the revelation of many new facial wrinkles as the pounds disappeared. My excess fat had always concealed them. My newfound wrinkles are part of my new identity, and I'm comfortable with that. Wrinkles don't destroy health. Obesity does. I've earned every one of those wrinkles in the battle of life and wouldn't trade them for excess pounds!

Although my waistline has never been dainty (currently thirty-two inches at 130 pounds), I have no problem accepting my expanded waist as that of a fit and healthy grandmother who once gave birth to a ten pound baby and is headed toward her sixties in a better-nourished body. It must be true that waistlines increase with age because mine expanded significantly. My waist is now a good five inches wider than it was at the same weight forty years ago, but I'm comfortable with myself. A "fluffy" waistline is easy to conceal under loose-fitting tops and styles that don't emphasize that part of my anatomy. I opt for elastic or stretch waistbands with room to breathe and avoid the hip-hugger pants that have become the latest fashion fad. I'm celebrating the new me as that of a maturing woman who has nothing to prove to anyone but herself.

Final hip and bust measurements minimized to a respectable range in the thirties.

A huge burden has not only been lifted from my body but also from my mind and spirit. Having struggled with the weight issue all my life, I have now achieved my weight goal, but it will still take continuous vigilance to hold my position. I need to fend off well-meaning friends or co-workers who shove dessert in my face and tell me that one piece won't hurt me. I realize their offerings are well intended, but they do not appreciate the hell of an addiction. During holidays, gifts of chocolates or cookies appear out of nowhere on my office desk. Co-workers may insist on offering the traditional slice of birthday cake and don't understand when the honored individual doesn't indulge. I either pass these sweets to a different area of our very large company, or I bury them in a trash bin. I no longer have any qualms about trashing something that is not nutritionally sound, but to spare hurt feelings, I do it out of sight of those who wished to honor me.

One must also remain vigilant to keep snacking to a minimum to avoid weight gain. If alcoholic beverages, potato chips, or crackers are a problem of excess for you, keep them out of reach. Avoid "carb creep." Empty calories add up and put on excess pounds. Any food that lacks nutrition and fiber can keep you eating mindlessly. Your body is screaming for foods with substance. When it is not satisfied, it will continue giving you hunger signals. The choice is yours whether you will continue eating "dead foods" that cause you to overeat or nutritious foods that fill you up and satisfy your appetite.

Some people may not want you to succeed where they have failed. Certain individuals may never be willing to put the time or effort into even trying to understand why you are abstaining from "dangerous substances to your health." They may feel threatened by your success. Obviously, becoming fit or healthy is not a priority for the whiner.

We need to make our homes safe houses where our children grow from good nutrition and develop healthful eating habits. We need to expose them to many different kinds of fruits and vegetables and a variety of nutrient-packed main dishes while they are growing. Many American children in this new millennium have never tasted a vegetable other than French fries or tomato paste on pizza. Their parents may want to blame the fast-food industry for making their children fat, but parents are responsible for what their pre-teenage children are eating.

At our house we keep many kinds of raw whole fruits on hand. My son-in-law likes to experiment with foods and prepares fabulous meals. My daughter blends healthy fruit shakes for the children after school. We peel oranges and slice apples and kiwi for them. They eat cherries and grapes for snacks.

You will find that you will actually spend less money on food if you are eating fewer processed foods and instead eating more fruits and vegetables. Processed and prepackaged food cost big bucks. You are paying quantities of money for the colorful packaging and for the convenience of someone else mixing the ingredients.

Children who drink low-fat milk and orange juice with real fruit instead of highly sugared and dyed fruit drinks and sodas will have considerably fewer colds, sore throats, and runny noses. Your children will eat what you eat. If all they have available is healthy foods, they will eat it when they get hungry enough. They learn by example.

When was the last time that you sliced up an apple for yourself? When was the last time you ate a handful of grapes or cherries? One of the fun things my grandchildren and I like to do in summer is eat cherries. We spit the seeds over the deck banister. It's all part of healthy memories we're instilling in our children. Summer and seed spitting go together in their minds.

Somewhere along my weight loss journey, I began writing this book to offer encouragement to others needing this information. I knew it would take time to complete my weight goal, and I wanted to use my time effectively to mark each achievement. The moment I broke the sugar addiction, I immediately experienced victory over mastering this issue. I never doubted that I would continue losing weight and eventually reach my goal of 130 pounds while eating a completely satisfying variety of nutritious foods. I know I keep repeating that you should not allow yourself to get too hungry, but women in our country have been brainwashed to starve themselves and think that by doing so they will lose weight. Your metabolism slows to conserve energy when you starve yourself.

After you have lost a large amount of weight, you may notice that your weight loss slows considerably. There is nothing wrong with you. Realize that it takes fewer calories now to maintain your current weight. Without excessive sugar, your appetite should also drop in acknowledgement of the lesser need for calories. You are not in a race to lose weight. Take whatever time necessary to lose your excess poundage and develop that healthier lifestyle. Relax and enjoy the journey. Don't set weight-loss goals that are impossible to achieve or maintain.

A huge milestone passed when 150 appeared on my scales for the first time in over twenty years and the dial pointed straight up and down. By that time, size twelve was working its way into my wardrobe. The pounds continued to dissolve until 130 arrived for the first time in over forty years. It was such a relief to finally achieve a goal that took all of my adult life to accomplish.

Do I miss chocolate, or am I ever tempted to eat something sweet? Since the craving cycle was broken, it is no longer a strong enough temptation to cause more than a passing glance. My body no longer screams for it, and I don't wish to return to that vicious cycle of cravings. I wouldn't trade my health or size now for where I was headed. I can actually enter an ice cream store with my grandchildren now and treat them occasionally, without being tempted to indulge myself.

Many times before, I gave up sweets for a few days but never long enough to break an addiction cycle. I had not fully comprehended that my problem stemmed from a sugar addiction. I didn't know why I was hungry all the time. I didn't understand the cravings could disappear and that without sugar my appetite would decrease. I was deceived into believing desserts were one of my biggest enjoyments in life. I didn't know that there would come a time when I would not even miss sugar or chocolate or desserts.

We are the first generation to see the quick destruction of our health because of the massive fast-food industry and unhealthy products devoid of nutrition that have been dumped on our society. We cannot walk down an aisle of our megasupermarkets without having thousands of choices of soft drinks, candy, donuts, ice cream, cakes, pies, and cookies screaming to us in all their colorful packaging. We must lay the blame squarely on our own poor choices. We are like children in a candy shop without restraints. We no longer need to work to prepare our food. We don't generate any physical activity to grow our food, harvest our food, preserve our food, or even cook our food.

We have swallowed the doctrine of "eat anything you want and eat it now" mentality, without a thought or care as to how it is directly affecting our health. We might mistakenly believe that a magic diet pill will cover up our own foolish choices and make everything all right again. Let me be the first one to break the news to you: a magic diet pill will not give you health. If you are not making healthy food choices, **no diet pill will prevent you from developing cancer, heart disease, type two diabetes, and overall poor health from terrible eating habits.**

Maintenance and Carb Creep

After achieving your weight goal, it continues to take some effort to maintain. If you are not vigilant, the pounds will creep back. The high-glycemic index foods must be kept to a minimal part of your diet, or you cannot hope to maintain. Have you started eating too many bread products again? Are you eating high-carbs often (chips, crackers, pasta, bread)?

Notice what you are eating, and adjust yourself accordingly.

No Eating After Dinner

Eating is habitual, and you must find what habits trigger you to overeat. After dinner I tended to graze. When the kids wanted snacks in the evening, I would help myself as well. This caused a constant flow of unnecessary calories and made it difficult to maintain my weight goal. After realizing the depths of my depravity, I changed. Now I eat dinner as soon as I arrive home from work and deny myself any further snacking until the next morning breakfast. The only substance allowed after dinner is water. For me, any munching after my evening meal is habitual and unnecessary. My body is not hungry, and I'm merely doing it because I happen to be in the vicinity of food.

Change Your Life to Change Others

Be the first wave of sugar abstainers who have decided that life will go on without that destructive substance in your life. Let's blaze a trail for others to follow. I believe the time is coming when more doctors will recommend total abstinence from sugar-infested products to help their diabetic and obese patients regain control over their health. Many doctors' voices are already singing to this tune.

Let's make such an impact on our society that more manufacturers will be willing to make healthier products without sugars in any hidden form, and society as a whole will become better informed as to the health dangers of sugar addiction. We have forgotten how to enjoy the natural taste of real food without sweeteners. We are dooming our children to sugar and poorer health by addicting them in infancy with baby foods and formulas that are loaded with unhealthy sweeteners.

Take your life back! Another three years will pass whether

or not you give up sugar, and you may become even heavier and less healthy than you are today. How would you like to turn the clock backwards, restore health, and escape from obesity? I did!

Chapter 14

Gastric Bypass Surgery

"Let me get this straight. You're operating on two
perfectly functioning organs to do what?"

BECAUSE WE LIVE IN a country where we like quick fixes, I felt
this subject was too important to ignore. If you are considering gastric bypass surgery, you need to be informed. It is not
"nirvana" or that state of total bliss, harmony, and peace forever. If you think that gastric bypass surgery is going to solve
all your obesity or health problems and leave you slim and free
of all weight-related symptoms from now to eternity, you are
misinformed. Gastric bypass surgery is very delicate and can
be deadly. It also does ***not*** guarantee weight loss. As the public
has become more aware of the possible benefits, the demand
has gone up and more inexperienced surgeons are performing
these operations. If the surgeon is less experienced, the likelihood of the patient suffering serious complications increases
quite significantly.

Let's say you pick an experienced surgeon, one who never
makes mistakes and does a perfect job on you. Are you really
going to lose the weight and keep it off? After all, isn't that
why you're willing to spend up to $45,000? Many insurance
companies will not cover this procedure, and as the risks and
complications become better known, even fewer of them are

willing. You believe that you will lose your obesity and keep it off, but is that true? You want all the weight to magically disappear and never come back. Otherwise, what is the point of going through the cost, pain, and long, slow recovery process of surgery? Have you even thought about the large percentage of other surgeries that many patients need after the bariatric surgery? Has anyone guaranteed to you that this will solve all of your obesity problems and henceforth and forever more, you will be free from obesity? Isn't this why you are going through all this time, effort, cost, and pain?

As obesity skyrockets, surgery that promises to solve obesity seems like the answer to prayer. The ads, unfortunately, seem to sway people into finding outcomes as positive, when there are serious risks that should carefully be weighed (no pun intended), as well as outcomes that are less than hoped for.

The surgeon begins with an incision into the upper abdomen to gain entrance to your stomach. Using a band, your doctor will section off the stomach where it meets the esophagus, creating a much smaller area for food to pass through that can hold anywhere from one to three ounces. In a bypass, the surgeon disconnects the small bowel and connects the larger portion of the intestine to the new stomach pouch. Have you ever considered what surgery shock does to your flesh or how long it really takes to recover from this type of major internal invasion and rearranging the plumbing of a perfectly designed body?

It's important to note that this surgery is drastic and is only a consideration for the morbidly obese, the definition of which is still being argued. It should not be viewed as a shortcut for someone struggling to lose less than one hundred pounds (although as its popularity grows, doctors will be compelled to tap further into the potential wealth in this area as long as there are customers willing to pay). **Since the surgery should only target candidates with one hundred or more pounds of excess weight, most patients approved for surgery will likely have**

other serious health risk factors going on that increase the surgery risk. Obesity, as you know, contributes to the likelihood of hypertension, type two diabetes, and pulmonary problems, all issues that can greatly affect the risk associated with any surgery.

While many candidates for bariatric surgical procedures already have joint issues, arthritis, and circulatory and respiratory problems because of poor-diet-caused extreme weight, the stomach and the small intestine are often working quite well. **Bariatric surgery cripples two fully functional organs: the stomach and the small intestine.** Since most absorption normally occurs in the small intestine, the risks of malnutrition or nutrient deficiency are very real. If you thought your body wasn't working well before the surgery, why would operating on two perfectly functioning organs and rearranging them in a manner in which they were not designed, make you think that your body will perform better after surgery?

Complications from bariatric surgery can and too often result in:

- Gastric juices and digests spilling into the abdomen (you can die from that).

- Peritonitis (a potentially fatal abdominal infection that can kill you).

- Nausea and vomiting (I never did enjoy that).

- Dehydration (which causes extreme weakness so you can't enjoy life, but what the heck, you'll lose some weight).

- A dumping syndrome when stomach contents move too quickly through the small intestine. This can result in violent vomiting and diarrhea, chronic nausea, weakness, sweating, and an inability to eat sweets with unpleasant or serious consequences.

- Weakening of bone can be the result of decreased absorption of calcium (so you may lose all that weight to have your bones weaken and end up permanently in a wheelchair).

- Infections where incisions have occurred.

- Gastrointestinal leaking.

- Connection site narrowing.

- Blood clots to the lungs (people die from those).

- Bowel obstruction (people die from toxemia).

- Bleeding and further infection (we're talking high-risk surgery).

- Spleen injury

- Iron deficiency resulting in anemia and other severe nutritional deficiencies. (If you think you can just take more vitamins to remedy the problem, remember that your body at this point is less able to absorb.)

- Gallstones (very painful, which leads to another surgery).

- Additional surgeries to address future complications.

- Hair loss and skin problems due to malnutrition from lack of absorption of nutrients.

- Death (and you thought being overweight was challenging)!

I have purposely avoided including bariatric "success" stories because I wish to provide some balance on this subject. Much of the information the general public comes across is slanted marketing, and when surgery is advertised, the risks will be minimized. I don't want anyone considering bariatric surgery to blindly believe that this surgery is a miracle cure or that the risks are minimal. In reality, it appears that significant weight loss is only achieved in less than half of the patients, **and a large percentage of them regain much of their weight**.

Are you willing to undergo a drastic surgery that cannot guarantee permanent weight loss? The surgery doesn't allow the metabolism or digestive system to operate optimally. **After several years, a majority of patients regain their weight** and feel helpless because their options are extremely limited and they are often in poorer health. As their health deteriorates, they often will seek additional surgical procedures with even greater risk to their health.

Bariatric patients are surprised to find that they have to constantly watch what they put into their mouths. They all fear regaining the weight. Some find it difficult to choke down the oversized nutritional pills and deal with all the abdominal cramping, loss of energy, and waves of nausea.

Some of the patients who are satisfied with the result and say they are happier since the surgery have mentioned undesirable aftereffects such as hair loss, bad breath, gum and dental issues, and severe vomiting if they take in more food than recommended.

Bariatric surgeries are increasing rapidly every year, as the demand for the surgery is so great that many hospitals have year-long waiting lists. In this environment, many surgeons wish to learn the techniques to treat a patient population that is desperate for help, and unethical practices will appear.

Long-term consequences remain uncertain.

Along with celebrity media hype, many patients are pleading for the surgery, not realizing that some of these "famous" patients have already regained much of their weight.

Can the surgery possibly even come close to meeting that patient's expectations based on the bariatric surgeries that have already taken place?

Please refer to web sites such as webmd.com and remedyfind.com/rm-3918-Gastric.asp or the Bariatric Surgery Registry for the latest studies and information regarding this hot topic.

CHAPTER 15

When It's Something Else

"When it still isn't working, keep searching."

THIS CHAPTER IS FOR those of you who have forsaken the sugar, thrown out the junk foods, exercise consistently, carefully monitor your eating habits to avoid too much bread or starches, and are still not losing weight. Possibly, you are even gaining. It could be something else. This chapter discusses some other possible causes of weight gain. Be honest with yourself and take responsibility for your own health. If doctors have checked you over and tell you it's all in your mind, keep searching. Read every medical journal (which you can check out from your local library for free), watch every medical documentary, and ask questions of every knowledgeable medical expert, until something clicks that is common to your problem. Use the Internet as a tool to track down illusive symptoms that aren't common to other people. Don't let a doctor tell you that there is nothing wrong, when your own body is telling you that something isn't right. Get informed.

Hyperthyroidism

Have you had your blood checked for thyroid hormone levels recently? My daughter at thirty-two years old was meticulous about what she ate, and no matter how hard or how often she exercised, she still wasn't losing weight. Then she discovered that she had low thyroid hormone levels in her blood. It seems that this is a very common malady, and without proper medication you can develop goiters and eventually blow out your pituitary gland while it's trying to overcompensate for the loss of the thyroid hormone. It took another year or two to get her medication stabilized to the point where she could lose weight again.

Children's weight problems are often directly linked to an underlying medical condition such as a sluggish thyroid. More women than men suffer from hypothyroidism, a condition in which the body produces too little metabolism-boosting thyroid hormone. A blood test can determine if this could be causing your weight woes. If it is, medication can help repair your metabolism.

Hypothyroidism is a condition where the thyroid gland does not produce enough thyroid hormone for whatever reason. Without this hormone, the body cannot function properly, **resulting in weight gain**, poor growth if it occurs in a child, slow speech, lack of energy, hair loss (which might also be a result of low protein levels), dry, thick skin, and increased sensitivity to cold. Have you been adding a sweater lately or wrapping up in more blankets when everyone else is too hot? If after reading this you suspect you might have this problem, get yourself checked. It's an easy test, and there are home kits available from your local pharmacy for hypothyroidism if you want to determine whether or not it's worth a trip to the doctor's office.

Those of you who do take thyroid medication and find it extremely difficult to lose weight may want to check out the book *The Thyroid Diet* by Mary Shomon. Your body cannot metabolize large amounts of carbs and fatty proteins. It may help you understand how your body is functioning at this point and how to counteract the negative aspects of weight gain.

Polycystic Ovarian Syndrome

While many of us have never heard of polycystic ovarian syndrome, it's actually one of the leading causes of infertility. **This disease is almost always associated with insulin resistance and weight gain**, a condition that makes it difficult for your body to process insulin. Eventually, your ovaries become overwhelmed, stop releasing eggs, and form tiny cysts instead. The symptoms are irregular periods, **diet-resistant obesity**, acne, excessive hair growth, and skin tags (tiny flaps). If your periods are chronically irregular or you develop any of the other symptoms, see your gynecologist.

Keep Searching and Ask Questions

For that small percentage of you who remain obese despite your best efforts and with no symptoms of the aforementioned ailments, I urge you to keep searching for answers and don't give up. Don't beat yourself up mentally if you are doing everything right and still the pounds persist. Every creature on God's earth has a different chemistry and DNA, making you precious and unique. You have great worth in God's sight. Psalms 115:12 tells us, "His thoughts turn toward us continually." He is always thinking about you and how you are doing. God didn't make any junk. You may be on this Earth to find the answers to pave the way for others who need help. Keep searching, and don't ever give up your quest for better health.

You've been given the tools to conquer your sugar addiction in this book, and you can have all you hoped for without the dangerous side effects of surgery. You can also develop a healthy eating lifestyle, something you cannot hope to achieve after such drastic surgery. Bariatric bypass surgery will assure that you will never eat normally again for as long as you live.

For the sugar addict, living without processed sugar is much easier than trying to control the amount of sugar that you allow yourself each day. I wish you health and the best life has to offer.

References Well Worth Reading

1. Atkins, Robert C. M.D., and Buff, Sheila. *Age-Defying Diet Revolution* (2000). St. Martin's Press, 175 Fifth Ave., New York, New York 10010.

2. Balch, James F., MD and Phyllis A., C.N.C. *Prescription for Nutritional Healing* (1997). Avery Publishing Group, 375 Hudson St., New York, NY 10014-3658.

3. Barefoot, Robert R. *Death by Diet* (2002). Triad Marketing, P.O. Box 590, Southeastern, PA 19399-0590.

4. Barefoot, R. R., and C. J. Reich, M.D. *The Calcium Factor: The Scientific Secret of Health and Youth* (2002). Triad Marketing, P.O. Box 590, Southeastern, PA 19399-0590.

5. Dadd, Debra Lynn. *The Nontoxic Home & Office* (1992). Jeremy P. Tarcher, Inc. 5858 Wilshire Blvd., Suite 200, Los Angeles, California 90036. Distributed by St. Martin's Press, NY.

6. DrNatura.com Inc., 6981 Curtiss Avenue, Sarasota, FL 34231. *Colon Cleansing, Constipation, Parasites*, IBS-On line Resource at http://www.drnatura.com.

7. Eades, Michael R., and Mary Dan, M.D., *The Protein Power Lifeplan* (2000). Creative Paradox LLC, Warner Boos, Inc. 1271 Avenue of the Americas, New York, NY 10020.

8. Geelhoed, Glenn W. M.D., and Barilla, Jean M.S. *Natural*

Health Secrets From Around the World (1997). Keats Publishing, Inc., 27 Pine Street (Box 876), New Canaan, CT 06840.

9. Heller, Dr. Rachael F, and Dr. Richard F. *The Carbohydrate Addict's Diet* (1991). Penguin Books, 375 Hudson Street, New York, New York 10014.

10. *Prevention Magazine.* Rodale Inc., 733 Third Avenue, New York, New York 10017.

CPSIA information can be obtained at www.ICGtesting.com
Printed in the USA
BVOW071414240512

291035BV00001B/78/A